Henrietta Wells has been practising homoeopathy for many years. She grew up familiar with homoeopathy because her godfather used it very successfully for treating his farm animals; neighbouring farmers would take his advice about homoeopathy in preference to that of the local vet. She became very interested in nutrition, including vitamin and mineral therapy, acquiring knowledge she uses when necessary in her practice. However, her experience of homoeopathy demonstrated that it could cure even where other therapies failed and led to her increasing interest in it. A great deal of her homoeopathic knowledge was gained from the renowned homoeopaths the late Dr. Margery Blackie C.V.O. and the late Dr. Charles Elliott in the 1970s. Dr. Elliott went out of his way to encourage her to become a professional homoeopath so she began practising in London and studied at the College of Homoeopathy. In 1987 she moved to Wiltshire in south-west England, where she has a flourishing practice with people coming from all over the UK and abroad to see her. In 1993 her first book *Homoeopathy for Children* was published. *Homoeopathy: The Modern Prescriber* is based on this but has been expanded to cover homoeopathic treatment for acute diseases for everybody whatever their age. When she has time she runs homoeopathic classes and gives talks, and she also gives homoeopathic tutorials to students.

Homoeopathy
The Modern Prescriber

Henrietta Wells
MCH, RSHom

WATKINS PUBLISHING
LONDON

This edition published in the UK in 2002 by
Watkins Publishing, 20 Bloomsbury Street,
London, WC1B 3QA

Cover design and illustration by Echelon Design
Designed and typeset by Echelon Design
Printed and bound in Great Britain by NFF Production

British Library Cataloguing in Publication data available

Library of Congress Cataloguing in Publication data
available

ISBN 1 84293 027 3

CONTENTS

CONTENTS

Appendices   *211*

Index   *217*

PREFACE

The media often refer to particular diseases as being 'incurable', yet I and other homoeopaths are often consulted by patients who have those very same conditions, and who are well on the way to recovery once they have started homoeopathic treatment. It is so sad that people do not realize homoeopathy could help them and that they do not have to put up with so much unnecessary suffering. It is quite surprising how little people know about homoeopathy. Some people think it is similar to herbalism or to do with nutrition and diet; sadly some others are simply dismissive or condescending about it without actually knowing what it is; and others think it is only suitable for minor ailments and that it is essential to take 'proper' medicine for something serious. All such ideas are totally incorrect and invariably occur when people know little or nothing about homoeopathy or its philosophy.

This book covers only those acute ailments which can be dealt with quickly, easily and confidently by the layperson. It does not cover chronic and more complicated conditions because it would be better and safer if they were treated by a professional homoeopath. In chapter one I have explained what homoeopathic medicine is and have given a brief account of its history. I have also gone into considerable detail about the handling, care and use of homoeopathic remedies as I have found over the years that this is an area where there is a great deal of ignorance. I hope I have answered many of the questions people have about homoeopathy in this chapter. Chapter two deals specifically with accidents and injuries and explains how to use homoeopathy for many first aid situations, while chapter three covers common acute ailments such as fevers, coughs and colds, earaches, food poisoning, etc. Chapter four is solely concerned with preventing and treating the acute diseases of childhood, whether the treatment is for a child or an adult. Many people, quite rightly, have become more aware of the very serious long-term damage to the immune system from inoculations and are looking for an alternative.

This chapter tells you how to recognize, prevent and treat the acute childhood diseases, and when to seek help from a professional homoeopath for the more serious ones. Chapter five gives advice on the care of homoeopathic remedies when travelling, and includes some advice about how to reduce the risk of deep vein thrombosis when flying. It also covers malaria prevention and treatment because many people are very unhappy about current conventional preventatives; these are either no longer particularly effective or have very serious side effects. The final chapter is a short Materia Medica of the remedies used most often in this book.

I hope by this book not only to enable the more open-minded to experience homoeopathy in a simple and practical way, but also to lead them to a better understanding as to what it is. People will discover that homoeopathy is an all-encompassing therapy which can be used for many diseases, even those of a very serious nature. I hope to demonstrate that each one of us experiences disease differently and how our unique picture of symptoms is what leads to the choice of the homoeopathic remedy. I show that all disease and suffering are part of an ongoing process and never happen in isolation simply out of the blue. I also explain that any true cure usually includes the mind, emotions and feelings because they are a vital part of the whole when treating disease, and cannot be separated from the physical. The body acts as a kind of shock absorber by helping the conscious and unconscious mind to carry its load; the body absorbs some of our mental and emotional tensions and problems (both past and present) and works them off in physical symptoms if it can.

Since this is a very practical book dealing with people's health, the advice, as well as any warnings and all instructions, should be taken seriously and followed carefully. This is not said to be alarmist but to point out that many conditions can become serious if not treated properly; you need to be conscientious, sensible and level-headed. Many people, occasionally even some practitioners, let fear rule them, so they panic when something looks frightening or serious, immediately thinking that allopathic (conventional) medicine should be used; in such a situation you should turn to a professional homoeopath for help without delay. Homoeopathy practised properly, particularly in the hands of an experienced practitioner who truly understands its methods, philosophy and effectiveness, can deal with very unpleasant and even life-threatening conditions. Most of us homoeopaths have often been challenged in this way and know very well our own capabilities and limitations, as well as homoeopathy's capabilities and limitations. Where I have suggested in this book that you should consult a professional homoeopath please do so, as well as on other occasions if you are feeling uncertain about what you are doing. However, please remember that most of the homoeopathic treatment described in this book is quite simple. People recover so quickly when treated with homoeopathic remedies for acute ailments and accidents that you should find it very rewarding as well as exciting when you start using the remedies. If you follow the advice carefully you should save yourself, your friends and family from a lot of unnecessary suffering – so please don't be afraid to have a go!

Chapter One

A GENERAL INTRODUCTION TO HOMOEOPATHY

1. Why do people turn to homoeopathy?

People tend to turn to homoeopathy or other alternative therapies because they have tried orthodox medicine and it has either failed them completely or they have had to cope with unpleasant or serious side effects from the drugs. Others have felt tired and below par for many years (symptoms which often precede more serious conditions) but, despite many tests and sometimes unpleasant investigations, it has not been possible for a diagnosis to be made for them. Since homoeopathy treats the individual as a whole, rather than just the disease, it is possible to treat people successfully who are feeling very unwell, in pain, or with unpleasant symptoms, but for whom there is as yet no orthodox diagnosis. In this way homoeopathy can prevent the onset of many serious conditions. Many things contribute to disease: the toxic load we acquire through daily life, weaknesses and tendencies towards certain diseases which we may inherit, and all sorts of stresses both emotional and physical – all these result in the body's natural healing powers failing; the body runs out of the energy to heal itself and the homoeopathic remedy acts as a stimulus which boosts this energy and so assists in the healing process.

Homoeopathy literally means 'similar suffering' and is based on the law of treating like with like; this means that a substance which can cause a certain picture of symptoms in a healthy person will cure that same picture of symptoms when met with in a sick person. Homoeopathic remedies are made in a very special way which involves giving only a very minute dose of the substance. This means that the remedies are not addictive, and do not have side effects.

People react in different ways to the same illness and treating the whole person means that the homoeopathic remedy is chosen especially because it suits that particular individual; this means that there could be ten people with flu and they each would have a different remedy or sequence of remedies. This is because although they have the same diagnosis, their individual symptoms, their individual ways of coping with stress, their individual characteristics and personalities vary considerably.

It is often not realized that, since homoeopathy is holistic in its approach, homoeopathic remedies can also help with all sorts of emotional complaints and stresses such as grief, anger, jealousy, fears of all kinds, many inadequacies, worries, shyness and phobias to name only a few. If left undealt with, most of these negative emotions eventually become contributing factors in triggering off physical disease of some kind, and one of the joys of homoeopathy is that the remedies work on both levels; the emotional as well as the physical. With homoeopathic treatment patients' general health gets better as well as the disease, so that their quality of life improves. Any negative emotions, which may hold patients back from making the most of themselves as individuals, will be reduced or eliminated; people find themselves feeling much more energetic and their general outlook on life is happier and more positive.

2. What is homoeopathy and how did it all begin?

HAHNEMANN

Samuel Hahnemann, the founder of the formal therapeutic system of homoeopathy as it is known today, was born in Germany in 1755. He was a brilliant linguist and paid his way through medical school by doing scientific translations. After becoming a very successful doctor he became disillusioned with what medical practice involved at that time; he felt that many of the practices did nothing to cure and quite often speeded the death of the patient. As time went on Hahnemann became more and more horrified by these experimental, unscientific and 'trendy' methods, not just those for physical illnesses but also by the barbaric treatment of so-called mental patients. Eventually he gave up his practice and turned again to translating scientific books to earn his living. He did a great deal more than simply translate, however. He verified, corrected, and amplified the works, and he was much respected and admired by the medical profession at that time.

LAW OF SIMILARS

When Hahnemann was translating a *Materia Medica* by William Cullen (who was a well-known professor of chemistry at Edinburgh University) he thought Cullen's explanation as to why the medicine China (Peruvian Bark) was successful in the treatment of malaria was not only inaccurate but also rather absurd. China had been used to treat malaria for over 300 years and its effectiveness for cure in many cases was well known. As it was one of the few successful treatments at that time it was of great interest to Hahnemann. While unhappy with Cullen's theories, Hahnemann knew that there had to be an explanation as to why China was often curative. Consequently he did an experiment on himself which involved taking 'four drams daily of China for several days'. The symptoms Hahnemann developed as a result of taking the China were typical of malaria. It is assumed that Hahnemann tried this particular experiment because he had already noticed from his translations that the poisonings (recorded in the *Materia Medica*) caused by crude doses, resembled the typical symptoms of the diseases for which they were *successfully* prescribed. He therefore came up with the theory that a substance which can cause certain symptoms in a healthy person can also cure those same symptoms in a sick person. Hahnemann was aware that this was not a new idea; before and during his time the question of whether a disease should be cured by similars or contraries was often debated. Hippocrates, nearly 2000 years earlier, was aware of this law of similars; that is, a substance will cure similar symptoms to those it can produce.

The word 'homoeopathy' literally means 'similar suffering' and is based on the law of similars. The law of similars – *similia similibus curentur*, or 'what a substance can cause it can also cure' – occurs throughout nature. For instance an unpleasant smell can be destroyed by a stronger smell, not by loud music. You can drown a nasty noise by another noise, not by switching on a light. Experiments have shown that engine noises can actually be silenced by exactly mimicking the wavelength of the noise produced. Starlight is obliterated by the stronger light of daylight at dawn. Diseases only coexist when they are dissimilar. When they are similar they destroy each other (provided they are not interfered with). Once Hahnemann had made his discovery he then experimented with other drugs and substances on his family and friends, building up a comprehensive Materia Medica.

PROVINGS

'Provings', as these homoeopathic experiments are called, are made very painstakingly. Each substance is taken daily by healthy men and women (as well as by some controls taking a placebo). Provers are never told what substance they are taking. All symptoms produced are noted with meticulous care; those produced by all the provers actually taking the substance are what make up the proving. The *Homoeopathic Materia Medica* is a record of these provings, which were the first attempt of any kind in the medical world of formal drug testing and standardization. You only have to read a small section of any drug picture or proving in a *Materia Medica* to appreciate the meticulous care and observation required. (Side effects of allopathic drugs – drugs used in conventional medicine – are in fact provings. Very occasionally doctors deliberately use a particular drug to treat a patient with symptoms similar to that drug's side effects; in other words using the drug homoeopathically.) Homoeopathic provings are always done on people, not on animals.

POTENTIZATION AND THE MINUTE DOSE

When Hahnemann first began prescribing homoeopathically, that is prescribing a substance which can cause similar symptoms to the ones it is intended to cure, he came across a major stumbling block. He realized that the aggravation caused by giving a crude dose of the homoeopathic remedy could be dangerous. He also knew that diluting the remedy would simply make it weaker and less effective, so he developed the idea of succussion. This literally means very 'vigorous shaking' of the bottle containing the liquid remedy a particular number of times at *each* stage of the dilution. He discovered that the remedy's energy and power to cure increased with each dilution, *providing it was succussed at each stage as well.* This is so despite the fact that the substance very soon becomes so diluted that there is no single molecule of the original substance left. It is very important to appreciate this as some homoeopathic remedies when they are mother tinctures (that is, before they have been either diluted or succussed) are poisonous; but by dilution and succussion they are rendered non-toxic and simply cannot have side effects as all that remains is a specific pattern of energy. Homoeopathic remedies are mostly made from plants and minerals. By the process of dilution and succussion one is able to use substances which may in their original state have been poisonous, but have been rendered harmless by the dilutions and also curative because they have been diluted *and* succussed. The remedy has stopped being a possibly toxic material substance and has become a safe energy remedy with its own individual wavelength. Every substance radiates energy at its own particular wavelength, although most radiations are only measurable by extremely sensitive instruments. Succussion of a homoeopathic remedy imprints the wavelength of the particular substance into the liquid remedy. Experiments have shown that freezing liquid homoeopathic remedies results in unique crystal structures with each remedy retaining a particular recognizable pattern, just as each remedy has its own unique radiating wavelength. During illness the cells of the body function inefficiently and their radiating wavelengths alter. The altered wavelengths produced by ill health can only be cancelled by a remedy which is capable of producing similar wavelengths; that is, homoeo-pathically.

According to modern physics, matter shows either particle or wave-like patterns of probability or activity depending on the way it is viewed. This demonstrates the fact that matter is not simply solid. Subatomic particles have properties which are only definable and observable through their interaction with other systems, which in turn are interconnections between yet more systems. They have absolutely no meaning as isolated entities. Thus matter is not passive and inert as we have been inclined to imagine, but is vibrating with rhythmic patterns of energy. It is dynamic. Quantum physics shows that during the accelerated collision process of particles, material particles are created and destroyed and their mass is transformed into energy. These facts should help us understand how a homoeopathic remedy may work. The principle of colliding particles is used in the succussion of homoeopathic remedies. A straightforward dilution only makes a remedy weaker, but dilution *and* succussion release energy from the mass of the substance of the remedy into the liquid carrier.

Today orthodox medicine explains illness mostly as a breakdown of parts at a physical or chemical level. If this mechanistic view were in fact true we would all become diseased every time we were in contact with a disease agent. However, most of us most of the time are quite unaffected by all the viruses and harmful bacteria that are in and around us. We only become ill when our bodies are disposed and susceptible. We do not all get ill from disease agents all of the time. This means that disease cannot possibly be just chemical or mechanical, it has to be purely dynamic in origin. So in order to make a remedy totally homoeopathic it should not only be able to produce those symptoms it is intended to cure, but also it should be dynamic (that is potentized by succussion) just as illness is dynamic in origin. Through-out the centuries this dynamic energy has been given many names such as vital force, vital body, life force, vitality and others. Whatever we call it we cannot on reflection deny its existence, not only in ourselves but also throughout the whole natural world. Its power to create order and harmony is all around us. It is the life energy which animates and controls the whole human organism. Without it we are just a batch of chemicals which would decompose and die. Any illness originates on this dynamic plane, when the body's natural healing powers fail. The homoeopathic remedy acts as a stimulus to the healing process.

MIASMS

Hahnemann sometimes found that the administration of the *similimum*, or homoeopathic remedy, along with the removal of any obvious contributing causes to disease, did not always result in a cure. He thought that the symptoms in such cases were signs of a much deeper seated chronic disease. This is where his theory of miasms comes in. During conventional treatment the drugs given are chosen for their opposing effect, going contrary to the direction of the natural healing process. This results in the natural centrifugal activity, the natural outlet of disease, being suppressed. The cells of the body then function inefficiently and, as mentioned before, their radiating wavelengths are altered resulting in permanent changes in their vibratory pattern. This means that although the symptoms treated by conventional medicine may disappear and the patient appears to be 'cured', in fact the symptoms have been driven underground and in time a deeper seated disease will emerge. This change weakens and lowers the energy level of the vital force and the weakness can be passed from generation to generation. Conventional medicine accepts that tendencies towards certain diseases are familial or inherited; homoeopathy explains how and why this happens, and how it can be prevented in the future. We can inherit miasmatic weaknesses just as we can inherit our looks and other characteristics. The miasm is a weakness created by the disease symptoms being suppressed and driven back inwards rather than cured. To remove this block to permanent cure Hahnemann administered a potency of the particular disease product concerned. He found that subsequent prescriptions of the *similimum* resulted in permanent cure.

TOTALITY

The fact that matter is only definable by its interaction with other systems, and that these systems in turn are interconnected with yet more systems, indicates the basic oneness of the universe and that no piece can exist in isolation. Matter of all kinds appears as a complicated web of interconnections between the various parts of the unified whole. This concept of wholeness is just as important in homoeopathy. The patient must be treated as a whole – the totality of the symptoms should lead to the choice of the homoeopathic remedy; this includes mental, emotional and physical symptoms as well as looking at the patient in the context of his or her relationship to the environment and all external stresses, strains and influences. There is a vast difference between this and conventional medical treatment where attention is almost exclusively focused on just the part that has gone wrong, as though that part exists in isolation from the rest of the body, the person and the world.

What is known today as naturopathy is in fact part of the therapeutic system of classical homoeopathy founded by Hahnemann. It is part of the concept of treating the person as a whole, which includes taking into account all external and environmental influences. Hahnemann maintained that poor living conditions, damp, hunger, lack of fresh air and of light, dirt and overcrowding (which were all very common in his time) contributed to illness. As with his other ideas Hahnemann was ahead of his time in this respect. Today, while some of these factors still contribute to disease in the Third World, elsewhere the things that contribute to disease are usually rather different. Now they can be the toxic load acquired by overeating and drinking, as well as from faddy diets or living off junk foods; lack of exercise or even sudden hard exercise; aluminium and other additions to the water supply; allopathic and pleasure drugs; and all the hundreds of chemicals put on the land as well as the hormone growth promoters and antibiotics fed to cattle. There can also be the miasmatic weaknesses we may inherit, the pace of modern life, overstimulation and quite often the prolonged use of television and computer games, as well as the inability to adapt to change and cope with stresses. If any of these are contributing to the suffering of the patient they must be removed and avoided where possible in order to regain health. The patient who is coming for homoeopathic treatment must be prepared to reconsider and adapt aspects of his or her lifestyle in order to help remove the illness and achieve better health.

SINGLE REMEDY

The importance of prescribing just a single remedy, not a mixture of drugs which many allopathic prescriptions contained then as now, was emphasized by Hahnemann before he even started his homoeopathic practice. He said that accurate prescribing could only be accomplished by giving one substance at a time and perceiving its effects. The single remedy is even more important with homoeopathic prescribing, partly because the remedies are proved singly not as mixtures. For instance, the remedies Ferrum Metallicum and Phosphorus have separate provings and drug pictures of their own; and while the Ferrum Phos. drug picture has similarities to both of them, it also has a unique drug picture of *its* own. It is crucial to find one remedy that is as similar as possible in all essential aspects to the disease picture presented by the patient. The remedy is only changed as the picture presented by the patient changes.

SUMMARY

Homoeopathy involves treating the sick person with a remedy that would produce similar symptoms if given to a healthy person. Only those symptoms a substance can cause, can it also cure. The remedy should be potentized by a process of serial dilutions and succussion, so that it is safe for the patient to take and is also dynamic just as disease is dynamic in origin. The potency should match the energy level of the patient. The homoeopath's job is to take into account all the symptoms the patient has and to choose a remedy from the homoeopathic Materia Medica which can produce similar symptoms. The homoeopathic Materia

Medica is a record of all the provings or drug pictures of the remedies. The homoeopath should also try to remove all the causes and bad habits which may be contributing to the disease. Symptoms are not the sign of a morbific process (disease process) but of a curative process. They are the diseased person's efforts to maintain order within by pushing the disease out to the periphery; the symptoms are the end result, not the cause, of the disease. The homoeopathic remedy is an energy which is matched to that person's unique picture of symptoms and stimulates that person in his efforts to throw off the disease. Allopathic (conventional) prescribing works in the opposite way. Given in crude material doses, the allopathic drug is chosen because it produces opposite symptoms to those presented by the patient. If the patient has enough energy, he continues to try to throw off the disease despite the opposing medication. This is why many allopathic prescriptions frequently have to be increased in strength in order to suppress the symptoms completely. When this happens the presenting disease is eliminated but the level of disease has been driven inwards mutating into something else much more serious, for instance asthma following the suppression of eczema. The homoeopath does not need to know the diagnostic 'label' given to the patient; this can in fact lead the homoeopath away from seeing the uniqueness of the individual. While the homoeopath can treat the patient long before the disease is so bad that it can have a diagnostic 'label', the allopath, or conventional doctor, cannot even start to treat the patient until he has that 'label'. While the homoeopath looks at the patient as a whole and in relation to his environment, the allopath specializes more and more until there are experts on every part of the body but nobody capable of looking at the patient as a whole. Homoeopathy has stood the test of time and is based on sound, solid, unchanging, natural laws, which are neither trendy nor faddy, and it is safe.

3. The difference between Acute and Chronic Conditions

Acute Conditions

These always have a clearly defined beginning and end, such as a fever, a cold or a cough, food poisoning or sunstroke, and are the type of conditions covered in this book. It is important to understand that acute diseases are acute exacerbations of the underlying chronic disease in an individual. The vital force or energy, which we all possess, is constantly trying to prevent the inward march of chronic disease and to repair and maintain order within the body, protecting the innermost core and pushing disease out to the periphery. When it succeeds in doing this an acute episode will emerge. This is a good, not a bad thing, providing it is not suppressed and driven back inwards again. The future prognosis will be good if at this crucial stage homoeopathic remedies are used; the homoeopathic treatment stimulates the natural healing powers of the body by driving disease outwards. The individual as a whole emerges stronger having successfully driven out the disease, rather than weaker as when the disease has been suppressed by allopathic medicine.

Chronic Conditions

Chronic conditions treated by ordinary medicine, or left untreated in those who have little vitality, are recognizable by the direction they travel in; they go from a less important organ to a more important organ, from the exterior inwards and from below upwards. For instance if someone has a rheumatic condition you will often find that it starts at their knees and then travels to their hips, or it starts in their finger joints and then goes to larger joints. While chronic disease travels inwards the natural vitality of an individual is constantly trying to push chronic disease outwards and this is usually manifested by an acute episode of some kind. It is therefore particularly important not to suppress an acute illness, as that would mean going in the opposite direction to the natural healing energies of the body. It is always crucial not to suppress any discharges or eruptions as they are indications that the body is trying its best to throw out an acute illness, and to stop the insidious march inwards of chronic disease. A homoeopathic remedy at this stage acts as a stimulus to the vitality to complete a true cure, going along with the *natural* healing processes by pushing disease outwards. Conventional medicine at this stage nearly always goes contrary to the natural healing process and drives disease back inwards. The damage of suppression is always particularly obvious in the treatment of eczema; steroid ointments heal up the skin and then within a year or so the patient develops asthma - the disease has gone from the periphery, the skin, into the lungs. Similarly the suppression of a streaming nose during a cold is nearly always followed by headaches and bunged up sinuses. These are two typical and easily observable examples of suppression. It seems to occur almost invariably as a result of allopathic treatment, which mainly involves giving medication that produces opposing symptoms to those presented by the patient, thereby going contrary to the natural healing processes of the body. If you question people carefully who have only been treated by conventional medicine, you will usually find that the illnesses they have had during their lives have become progressively more serious, affecting more inner and more important functions of the body. The results of such suppression can occur either immediately or many years later. Chronic disease, as well as health, are both on-going living processes. A diagnosis implies that the particular disease just happened to occur at that particular time out of the blue, but there is always a past aetiology (cause of the disease) and some sort of future prognosis. The past aetiology may be miasmatic weaknesses (which if left untreated by homoeopathic remedies are passed on to the next generation), the toxic load of all kinds, negative thought or behaviour and many other contributing factors. The future prognosis depends on whether homoeopathy is used to help stimulate the body's natural healing vitality to throw off disease, or whether allopathic medication is used which will continue the suppression of the vitality, resulting in the disease's inevitable march inwards; this leads to even more serious complaints and more chronic disease. It is so important to realize that the way you treat yourself today reflects the health (or disease) that will affect you in the future and that the level of health you have today reflects how you (and your forebears) were treated in the past. The damaging results of suppression may well take some time to emerge but they will always do so in time.

4. Homoeopathy from childhood to old age

At every stage of life, as your children grow up and develop, all through their careers and into retirement and old age, you will find that homoeopathy can lend a helping hand. This can start with the use of Arnica to prevent any shock during birth and any bruising from forceps deliveries. During the first few months of life and onwards there are many acute ailments babies may get which you can learn to treat from this book. These may include such things as colic or teething problems; ear inflammations, infections and fevers. As the remedies work so quickly your child will be much happier and more content than he would otherwise have been, and you will be less likely to have to endure endless sleepless nights.

As your children learn to crawl and walk, and then, growing older, become more adventurous, there will inevitably be many accidents around the home and this is where you will find homoeopathy works so quickly that it will really surprise you. The accidents and injuries you can treat at home are in chapter two of this book. You will also find that you can help your family a great deal with homoeopathic remedies for acute ailments such as sore throats, colds and coughs, croup, food poisoning, headaches, flu, carsickness and nervousness before tests, exams or going to the dentist.

With acute conditions, you will find that your family recover much more quickly with homoeopathy than if they have conventional treatment. For instance, if one of you has acute earache from a middle ear infection and you are able to prescribe the correct homoeopathic remedy, there should be some immediate improvement and a decrease in pain within about ten to fifteen minutes (sometimes a lot less) followed by a complete cure within a few hours, or occasionally a day or two at the most. When homoeopathic remedies are used, the treatment works with the natural healing processes of the body and the disease is not suppressed. On the other hand, with antibiotics used to treat the infection, improvement will usually take much longer. With conventional treatment the condition often recurs until eventually, once there have been frequent enough suppressions with antibiotics, more serious chronic disease results (although this may only manifest itself years later). With homoeopathic treatment the patient will feel much better after than before the illness, whereas after conventional treatment there is often damage from side effects of the drugs used; these side effects may not always be very serious but they can be extremely annoying and tiresome, and can take a long time to shake off (such as thrush following the use of antibiotics).

Similarly, from a prevention point of view, the use of homoeopathy for acute ailments avoids much prolonged suffering. For instance, if someone begins to run a high temperature which could be the onset of a two to three week dose of flu and you prescribe the appropriate homoeopathic remedy, you will be able to nip the illness in the bud; there should be almost immediate improvement with all the symptoms usually disappearing within a few hours, or at the most within a day or so. Children usually tend to have a great deal of energy and for this reason they frequently respond to the homoeopathic remedies extremely fast which is very satisfying from the prescriber's point of view, particularly if you are an anxious parent wondering if you have given the correct remedy. It is wonderful to be able to help stop their suffering so quickly and efficiently.

One minor but quite practical consideration regarding young children is that they find that homoeopathic remedies taste nice and are perfectly happy to take them, even when small babies. Also the remedies are perfectly safe, so if by mistake your child manages to get hold of a remedy and eat the bottle-full, there should be no detrimental effects from the remedy. Another consideration is that, instead of hanging around in a crowded waiting room at your doctor's surgery, you can prescribe a homoeopathic remedy at home which should improve the condition in less time than you would have spent waiting to see your doctor. Children and adults, even if they have not been treated homoeopathically in the past, find the remedies enormously beneficial not just for physical problems but emotional ones as well. Those who have a need to talk and seek psychiatric help or counselling do extremely well when they combine this with homoeopathy; both therapies work together very well in such conditions as grief, post traumatic stress syndrome, addictions, and mental illness as well as for many other emotional or behavioural problems.

On a typical day I could find myself treating people with any of the following conditions: asthma, eczema and many other skin problems, bed-wetting, ulcers, warts, excessive nervousness or shyness, depressions, fears, phobias, panic attacks, temper tantrums, nightmares, behavioural problems, learning difficulties, dyslexia, digestive problems of any kind, ME, MS, psoriasis, hayfever, migraine, chronic headaches, sinusitis, fibroids, period pains and related problems, PMT and PMS, post-natal depression, sterility, menopause problems, prostate problems, diabetes, rheumatism, arthritis, emphysema, Parkinson's disease, epilepsy, allergies of many kinds, memory problems as well as a chronic tendency towards things such as fevers, swollen glands, tonsillitis, coughs, ear infections or cystitis and many other serious conditions.

If your family uses homoeopathic remedies for all their acute ailments throughout their life you should find that, since nothing has been suppressed by allopathic drugs over the years, they will be much less likely to succumb to the chronic diseases of middle age and old age. All the problems of menopause can be minimized or cured and even the very old respond wonderfully well to homoeopathic remedies. Amongst many other benefits, flu jabs become unnecessary, debilitating coughs improve rapidly, strokes following head injuries from falls can be prevented and broken bones from falls and accidents heal faster. Since homoeopathic treatment involves treating the whole person and the remedies are chosen according to an individual's characteristics, moods and personality, as much as for the physical conditions and modalities, you will find that as the patient gets better by using homoeopathic treatment there will invariably be a corresponding improvement in temperament. A clingy, weepy, over-shy person will become less so; a snappy, angry, impatient person will become more amenable and pleasant to have around, and so on. This is the case whether the treatment is for an acute or a chronic condition and an improvement in temperament is always an excellent sign; improvement in the physical condition will follow very soon if it has not already started.

Not forgetting the extremely beneficial role homoeopathic remedies can play in treating the acute childhood diseases (see chapter four), I think the main advantages of using homoeopathy for treating your family can be summarized as follows:

1. In acute illnesses, accidents and emergencies you will find the speed with which there is improvement quite surprising; many of my patients simply cannot believe how fast it can be. Since the improvement is so fast this also means that suffering is minimized.

2. Your family will have had no allopathic drugs, so there will have been no danger of side effects because homoeopathic remedies are extremely safe. Side effects from conventional drugs, even when not particularly serious, can none the less be extremely irritating and difficult to get rid of.

3. The acute illnesses will not have been suppressed because homoeopathic treatment goes along with the natural healing processes of the body. This is particularly important with regard to the acute childhood diseases (see chapter four). By avoiding suppression of disease and thence, at the very least, delaying the onset of serious chronic disease later on in life, homoeopathy has a vital preventative role to play. Middle and old age will be healthier and happier.

4. As your family are treated with homoeopathy and therefore no suppressions occur, you are in fact contributing towards a much healthier life for them in the future, not only in the short term but in the very long term as well. This does not only mean that they will have a lot less illness as they grow older, but also that mentally and emotionally they will be much happier and consequently be able to make the most of themselves as individuals. They will become contributors to, rather than takers from, the world in general. By the time your children become teenagers they will be much less likely to be bored, uncooperative or difficult; they will be more confident than

they otherwise might have been and therefore much less likely to succumb to peer group pressure to experiment with drugs, or indulge in any other destructive behaviour. With homoeopathic treatment life is happier, more complete, and there is much less suffering.

5. Answers to some common criticisms of homoeopathic medicine

Until recently one of the main criticisms of homoeopathy has been about the minuteness of the dose. It was considered absurd that the remedy could do anything at all, curative or otherwise, when there was no measurable quantity of the original substance left in it as a result of the dilutions. The importance of the succussions was ignored. However, the advent of modern physics (particularly the quantum theory) has now explained how matter involves movement and energy and is not simply inert as once thought. It explains the fact that the succussion part at each stage of the potentization process (which is so essential) *could* energize the remedy. Unfortunately the quantum theory seems to be very little understood generally and there are still some who run down homoeopathy because of the smallness of the dose.

There is now also a general awareness that in some way people's energy is a major factor in the healing process (although this is undetectable by technology) and therapies which involve stimulating this natural healing energy in some way (such as homoeopathy and acupuncture) are becoming more accepted. How the healing energy actually works is not well understood, although again modern physics does make it more comprehensible.

Another major criticism concerns proof and medical testing of homoeopathic remedies. The allopathic medical profession tests specific drugs for specific named diseases; this is fine if you are choosing the drug for that particular named disease. However with homoeopathy the practitioner is choosing a remedy based on the picture of the individual as a whole. Personality characteristics, general likes and dislikes of all kinds, all the physical details of the condition as well as any miasmatic weaknesses (see page 7) are the reasons a particular remedy is chosen. Even when treating simple colds or fevers (see pages 67–86), there are many remedies to choose from and the one which will cure depends on its similarity to how the patient is behaving and feeling, not on the disease label he has been given. As already mentioned, you could have a number of people with the same diagnosis and each person would be given a different homoeopathic remedy or sequence of remedies, because each one has a different personality, different characteristics, different modalities, miasms and so on, although they all have the same disease. No two people are exactly alike and for this reason it is impossible to test homoeopathy in the same way as allopathy, as it would deny the essential nature of what homoeopathy is – *choosing a remedy which is capable of producing symptoms in a healthy person similar to the specific picture of symptoms of a particular sick individual, and not chosen for the named disease.* However, all homoeopathic remedies are proved (see page 4) in great detail and homoeopaths know exactly what each remedy is capable of curing, providing it is similar to the case. In fact homoeopaths know about the remedies in considerably more detail than allopaths do from *their* manner of drug testing. It also appears to have been forgotten that it was Hahnemann who was the first person to introduce the idea of drug testing; it has merely been adapted to suit the allopathic medical profession. Discussions have taken place as to the various methods of conducting research and hopefully this will lead to research methods useful for homoeopathy.

When a patient under homoeopathic treatment starts recovering from a disease which is considered incurable by conventional medicine, some allopaths then deny their original diagnosis and say there must have been a mistake. This happens far too often to be explained by the odd mis-diagnosis. It seems extraordinarily short-sighted of those conventional doctors to deny the possibility that using another therapy could result in a cure. Some doctors will also express doubt about the diagnosis of one of the acute childhood diseases when, as a result of homoeopathic treatment, the symptoms become so mild that the child suffers little, if at all. Another comment, frequently made, attributes the success of homoeopathy not to the choice of the similar remedy, but to the fact that homoeopaths devote a great deal more time to their patients when they take a case than do ordinary doctors. Obviously time taken in talking through problems is an enormous help to those who are sick, but no amount of talk is going to bring down a raging temperature in a matter of minutes, if not seconds; no amount of talk is going to eliminate pain from a burn or other injury and start the healing process, again in a matter of minutes; no amount of talk will calm down and render pain-free in a few seconds a colicky, teething baby who is yelling in fury and pain - this list could go on forever. As far as chronic conditions are concerned the same applies: like all homoeopaths I treat people with serious illnesses (both physical and emotional) which they have had for a long time. Most of them have spent much time seeing specialists of various kinds and despite this their conventional treatment appears to have failed; many have sought psychiatric help or counselling as well and still have not improved. They then come to me, frequently in despair. Under homoeopathic treatment they do begin to feel and get better. How can their improvement possibly be put down to just talk and listening, particularly when they have already done that with conventional specialists, psychiatrists or counsellors? It is worth pointing out that as far as animals are concerned there is obviously no counselling or talk involved, yet they respond very well to homoeopathy.

This leads to the point about belief itself. Often it is remarked that if one believes in a particular therapy then one is more likely to be cured by it. While I am sure that hope and belief make an enormous difference in some cases, numerous patients do *not* believe they will get better and are remarkably cynical about homoeopathy, yet they *do* get better against all the odds. By the time patients turn to homoeopathy for treatment of chronic diseases they have generally been ill for quite a long time. They usually have had suppressive treatments (sometimes for years) and are therefore physically and emotionally much weaker than when they first became ill and sought conventional treatment. Many tell me they are sure that homoeopathy cannot help them but that someone in their family has bullied them into coming to see me. Despite all this, they do get better. While a positive outlook is of enormous benefit during the curative process, equally experience has shown that belief in a cure frequently plays no part at all in the process because belief simply is not there. Can your dog know whether it is being given an antibiotic or a homoeopathic remedy? How then can belief play an essential role?

6. Can one use homoeopathic remedies at the same time as taking allopathic medicines?

One of the main differences between homoeopathy and allopathic medicine is that homoeopathy builds up the general health of individuals, delaying or preventing the onset of serious conditions, increasing their energy to deal with acute conditions, giving hope and optimism and enabling them to move forward in their own personal development; whereas allopathic medicine concentrates on the disease, the diagnosis and the fear of the disease. There is a tendency to remove the disease at all costs, regardless of how the treatment may affect the well-being of the patient; the medication given produces opposing symptoms to those presented by the patient and thus goes contrary to the natural healing energies of the body. Homoeopathy is much gentler and safer, going along with and assisting the natural healing processes of the body.

Acute Conditions

Homoeopathic remedies do not interfere with allopathic medicine; it is perfectly safe to take homoeopathic remedies for the acute situation if you are also having to take allopathic medicines for some other chronic condition. On the other hand, allopathic medication for chronic conditions can make the homoeopathic remedy less effective although this is less likely during acute homoeopathic prescribing. When treating acute conditions with homoeopathic remedies it is not a good idea to give ordinary medicines at the same time for the *same* acute condition. This is because the unique symptom picture for which you are prescribing would then change and become unclear, making it hard to prescribe the remedy that is homoeopathic to the case. It is best to stick to one kind of treatment only for acute diseases.

Chronic Conditions

Allopathic medication for chronic diseases can make homoeopathic treatment for chronic disease less effective, but usually this homoeo-pathic treatment should decrease the need for allopathic medication until eventually it should not be needed at all. Depending very much on the individual, the disease, and the medication, some people can come off their drugs virtually at once while others must come off gradually. Either way treatment must be done under the supervision of the homoeopath and/or the doctor. If homoeopathic treatment for chronic ailments is to be successful it must be carried out by a professional homoeopath; it is a great mistake for the layperson to attempt this and can lead to a lot of disappointment and suffering. If it were an easy thing to do there would be no need for the long and thorough training which classical homoeopaths undergo.

7. How homoeopathic remedies are made

Hahnemann realized that some of the natural remedies he wished to use were potentially dangerous, but that simple dilution would render them ineffective. This is when he came up with the idea of potentizing or energizing the remedy by a process known as succussion (see pages 5–6). This literally means 'vigorously shaking' the bottle containing the liquid remedy at each stage of the dilution. Having made up the Ø, the symbol for the mother tincture (this is the original undiluted substance), the pharmacist mixes one drop of it with nine drops of alcohol and vigorously shakes, or succusses the mixture a specific number of times. This is now called the 1X. One drop of 1X is then taken and mixed with nine drops of alcohol and vigorously shaken, or succussed; this new mixture then becomes the 2X. This process is continued up to whatever potency is required. The same method is used when making centesimal potencies, only then ninety-nine drops of alcohol are used at each stage instead of nine drops. The remedy's energy and power to cure is *increased* with each series of dilution, provided it is succussed at *each* stage as well. The higher the potency is, that is the more diluted *and* succussed it is, the more potent and energetic it becomes. Therefore:

IX = 9 drops of alcohol and one drop of Ø, and succussed
2X = 9 drops of alcohol and one drop of IX, and succussed
3X = 9 drops of alcohol and one drop of 2X, and succussed
4X = 9 drops of alcohol and one drop of 3X, and succussed

and so on up as high a potency as is required. Also:-

IC = 99 drops of alcohol and one drop of Ø, and succussed
2C = 99 drops of alcohol and one drop of IC, and succussed
3C = 99 drops of alcohol and one drop of 2C, and succussed
4C = 99 drops of alcohol and one drop of 3C, and succussed

and so on up to 1M. X potencies are tenths, C potencies are hundredths, M potencies are thousandths. When a remedy name has just the number after it, 6 or 30 or whatever, it *always* is the centesimal potency; so when people refer to a 6 or a 30 they always mean a 6C or a 30C. Other potencies, for example the X or M range, that is tenths or thousandths, will *always* have the letter after the number. It makes no difference if the letters C, X, or M are written as capital letters or lower case. (In some European countries the letter D is used instead of X and cH or CH is sometimes used instead of C.)

Occasionally people in my homoeopathic first aid classes have completely misunderstood about potentization and think that taking five pills of a 6C would be the same as taking one pill of a 30C. If you are thinking like this as well it means that you are still thinking along the lines of material quantities, rather than dilutions and succussions producing an energy and potency. Please reread this chapter because it is essential that you understand this.

8. Rules about handling, care of, and taking homoeopathic remedies

As you will have realized from the previous section, homoeopathy involves giving a very minute dose indeed. For this reason it is very easy to spoil the remedies if they are mishandled. The remedies can even be spoiled by strong smelling or scented substances. It is best not to keep them in the bathroom or in the kitchen, nor anywhere where some inquisitive person may tamper with them without you knowing.

During the succussion process the remedies have to be in liquid form. This liquid is then used to medicate tablets, pills, pilules (small round sucrose pills), powders or liquid carrier. It does not matter in what form the remedies are taken; it is simply a question of which you prefer or find most convenient.

Here are some basic rules to follow:

1. Keep your remedies in a cool, dry, dark place, well away from any strong smelling or scented substances. Never open them in the kitchen where someone may be peeling onions or where there may be other cooking smells. Keep them well away from aromatherapy oils and scented soaps.

2. Pills and powders should not usually be touched by hand because any smells, even scented soap residue, could antidote them. Powders should be tapped into the centre of the paper and from there onto the tongue. Pills should be placed on the tongue direct from their bottle cap. If they are in an envelope use a teaspoon to remove a pill. Wash the teaspoon if you change to a different remedy. It is a good idea to have soft tablets or remedies in liquid form for babies as they are easier to administer, but if you only have pills or tablets you can crush a few between two teaspoons and give the baby the resulting powder. With liquid remedies put 2-3 drops into about a teaspoon of water and give that as the dose. If no water is available give it neat.

3. The remedy is not absorbed via the stomach or intestines but its energy is assimilated via the saliva. For this reason the tablet or powder should be allowed to dissolve naturally on or under the tongue. If a tablet is very hard it may be lightly crushed with the

teeth and then dissolved. A remedy in liquid form should be held in the mouth as long as possible before swallowing; do not worry too much about this when giving a liquid remedy to babies, as the remedy will usually have been in the mouth long enough by the time it will have taken them to lick their lips and swallow. The remedy should never be washed down.

4. A remedy should always be taken in a naturally fresh mouth. Do not take it within half an hour of eating, drinking, sucking sweets, chewing gum, smoking or cleaning the teeth. (This is particularly important in non-acute situations when only one or a few pills are given and the effectiveness is expected to last over a number of weeks or months. This is usually the case for long-term prevention of diseases and when consulting a professional homoeopath.) Many of my patients get overanxious about this aspect of taking the remedies during acute illnesses and emergencies. At such times it is best to give the remedy regardless; the chances are that when people are fairly ill they will not have been doing any of these things anyway. With regard to people drinking liquid during a fever, water is fine as it has no particular taste, only make sure they do not actually wash the remedy down with it; with stronger tasting things, once the taste of whatever it was has left your mouth for a few minutes, then it is probably OK to take the next dose of remedy if you need it. During these acute situations remedies are able to be repeated much more often than during treatment for chronic ailments (prescribed for by your homoeopath), so if one dose is spoiled by mistake it does not matter quite so much in an acute illness as you are able to repeat it whenever it is necessary.

5. Do not transfer remedies from one container to another; keep them in the container you buy them in, unless you are replenishing an old bottle, but it **must be for the same remedy and the same potency**. If you accidentally drop one or more tablets they should be thrown away and not put back into the bottle.

6. Certain substances antidote homoeopathic remedies in most patients. You must therefore avoid taking them internally or using them externally in any form for the duration of the treatment until

you are completely better. These are coffee, peppermint, menthol, eucalyptus, camphor, Olbas Oil, tea tree oil and frankincense oil. Remember that some of them can be included in many other products, such as in teas, sweets, cough sweets, lip salves, menthol cigarettes, chest-rubs, Vick etc. **It is particularly important to avoid these substances when you are doing long-term prevention with homoeopathy for any disease, as well as when having long-term constitutional treatment.**

7. Many brands of toothpaste contain mint. It is best to use a non-minted type if possible. Fennel is very good.

8. Avoid taking other medication for the same acute condition as this will distort the picture for which you are prescribing and make it difficult, if not impossible, to choose the homoeopathic remedy; and if you do not choose the similar remedy then the remedy will not work.

9. Never keep remedies close by a mobile phone that is switched on, as this can interfere with the action of the remedies. Care should be taken with any remedies that you keep with you in your pocket or bag. Some photographic shops and a company called TravelSmith (0800 783 3030) sell small lead lined bags (for films) which can be used to protect your remedies wherever you go.

9. Rules about taking the acute case and then choosing a remedy

When you decide to treat anyone in your family it is important to think about, notice and consider carefully *all the symptoms* that are unique to that individual at the time. Having done this, only then should you start trying to match this total picture of symptoms to a remedy. If you do not do it this way round (that is, matching the totality of symptoms to a remedy) it is probable that you would end up trying to match a remedy to the symptoms - and this usually results in matching a remedy to only *some* of the symptoms; the chances are that those symptoms would be the ones which most alarmed you and/or would be the most noticeable, with you usually missing out some very important details. If this happens it is very difficult to choose the similar remedy because you probably would choose a remedy which is only partially similar to the total picture of symptoms presented by the patient; with the result that the patient may not get better, or that improvement may be extremely slow. You must always *take the case first*, and *then choose the remedy*.

When taking the acute case the things to consider are:

Mentals

How is the patient behaving? How would you describe the behaviour? Is he restless, fearful, angry, violently angry, grumpy, shocked, dazed, or what? Is he better or worse for being alone; clingy or more irritable if you pay him attention; does he grumble or make a terrific fuss at every noise or at anything in particular that you do?

These are just a few general ideas to help you notice how the patient is behaving. If you are already irritated by him yourself do not exaggerate his behaviour; alternatively if you love him dearly do not be blind to his bad temper or whatever negative behaviour he is showing. Do not be critical; you must simply observe and record the symptoms so that you can choose the similar remedy, accepting that this is how he is behaving at this particular time and it simply indicates what remedy is needed.

Generals

This is a list of important things to notice if they affect the patient *generally as a whole*, rather than just affect any particular part:

The *time* when he is better or worse, or when the acute illness began.

The *speed* of the onset of the illness; quickly, over a matter of hours, or slowly over a few days.

The *position* the patient is most comfortable in; the position that makes him worse.

Whether he is better or worse for *motion*.

His colouring and *appearance*; flushed, pale, changeable or anything else.

His reaction to *temperature*; to hot or cold food or drink; to being covered or uncovered; to hot or cold applications.

His reaction to *weather*; if he is worse for draughts; the kind of weather it was when the illness began; if he was exposed to extreme heat, cold, wet, wind, sun, or if it was dry.

His reaction to *light or dark*.

Whether one *side* is worse than another, or if this chops and changes.

If there are any *discharges*; if so what colour they are, whether bland, irritating, profuse, itchy, thick, thin, slimy, sticky or lumpy.

Appetite; if the patient desires anything in particular, or if he is made better or worse by anything in particular.

Thirst; for large quantities, for sips, for nothing, for what kind of drinks, for hot or cold drinks.

Pains; what they feel like, where they go.

Touch/pressure; whether this makes things better or worse.

Whether or not the patient is *sweating*; where he is sweating, if he is better or worse for sweating.

Particulars

These are the symptoms which only affect a *particular part* of the patient rather than the patient as a whole. The above modalities should be considered again but only in relation to the particular part of the body affected.

This list may seem rather daunting but on the whole the patient will tell you or it will be fairly obvious to you what the symptoms are in any acute case. This list is just to help you appreciate the kind of things to look out for so that you can build up a total picture of symptoms to enable you then to differentiate between one remedy and another. There will nearly always be at least three, but probably a lot more, very noticeable symptoms. It is often a good idea to spend a minute or two writing down all the symptoms which the patient is presenting, observing the patient carefully and checking through the above list to make sure you have not missed anything.

When taking an acute case certain symptoms carry more weight

Remedy Analysis Chart

NAME											DATE										
1.											6.										
2.											7.										
3.											8.										
4.											9.										
5.											10.										
Remedy	1	2	3	4	5	6	7	8	9	10	Remedy	1	2	3	4	5	6	7	8	9	10
Acon.											Hyper.										
Ailanth.											Ignatia										
Allium-c											Ipecac.										
Ant-c.											Kali-bi.										
Ant-t.											Lathyr.										
Apis											Lach.										
Arg-n.											Lac-c.										
Arnica											Ledum										
Ars-a.											Lyc.										
Arum-t.											Mag-p.										
Bellad.											Merc-c.										
Bell-per.											Merc-s.										
Bryonia											Nux-v.										
Canth.											Opium										
Calend.											Parotid.										
Carbolic.											Ph-ac.										
Caul.											Pertus.										
Caust.											Phos.										
Cham.											Phys.										
China											Phyt.										
Cimic.											Pilocar.										
Cina											Podo.										
Cocc.											Puls.										
Coff.											Pyrog.										
Coloc.											Rhus-t.										
Cuprum											Rumex										
Diphther.											Ruta										
Drosera											Silica										
Dulc.											Spong.										
Euphr.											Staph.										
Eup-per.											Stram.										
Ferr-p.											Sulph.										
Gels.											Symph.										
Glon.											Tetanus										
Hep-s.											Vespa c.										
Hyos.																					

than others. As a general rule the Mentals are more important than the Generals and the Generals more important than the Particulars. However, if a General or Particular is very unusual then it would become more significant. For instance, if someone has a burning pain which is better for heat that would be more unusual and therefore more important a symptom than a burning pain better for cool. Similarly, if a symptom is very intense then it carries more weight than if it is not. At this stage it is helpful to rewrite your list of symptoms in order of importance. Now that you have a clear total picture of symptoms you should start looking through the appropriate section in this book to find the most similar remedy. You may now wish to use the Remedy Analysis Chart across to help clarify the symptom picture.

You could copy this chart and use it when you are working out what remedy to take. The top few lines are so that you can list the symptoms unique to the patient at that time. The rest of the chart is a list of the remedies in this book and the ten numbered columns refer to each of the ten listed symptoms above them. The purpose of this is to make the choice of homoeopathic remedy easier.

When you have written down all the important unique symptoms for the patient, you then rewrite the list of symptoms in order of importance. You then should list these symptoms here in the chart starting with the most important as number 1, going up to as many as number 10 if you have them. The next job is to mark off in column number 1 all the remedies which have that symptom. You do the same for symptom number 2 and so on until you have charted all the main symptoms. Obviously you do not have to have as many as 10 symptoms but the more you do have, provided they are unique to the patient, the better. *You do not put down the symptoms that everyone would have for the condition, but only the ones which are peculiar and unique to that particular person.* You will then see that certain remedies are much more strongly indicated than any others. You should check those remedies in the Materia Medica in chapter six and in the appropriate chapters for the condition concerned. Reading more about the particular remedies in the different sections will help you get a better feel and understanding about them, thus enabling you to choose the right one. The remedy that covers *the greatest number of the most unique or most strongly indicated symptoms*, should be the one that is most homoeopathic to the case, and the one that should result in cure. All this may seem rather slow and laborious but it will help you learn how to prescribe; you will be more likely to be detached and less likely to make mistakes. It is a very good way of organizing the information you get from the patient so that you can build up a good symptom picture. It will also help you learn more about the remedies and make you think more clearly during acute prescribing.

10. *Rules about dosage, potencies and repetition of doses*

A GENERAL INTRODUCTION TO USING POTENCIES

When choosing a potency there are two main considerations:-

1. The potency has to match the energy level of the patient. You should always start by giving the remedy in a low potency, a 6C, unless the patient is very 'energetically' ill, such as being extremely restless or tossing and turning a lot in bed. In this case you should consider starting with a higher potency, such as a 30C; or else be aware that you may have to change to a higher potency fairly soon if the 6C does not hold. People who are very elderly and/or low in energy due to illness, are unlikely to need a 30 to start off with, and will respond better if you start with a 6.

2. The potency has to relate to the location of the disease. By this I mean that you should consider where the emphasis of the most important symptoms lies - whether this is more on the emotional level or more on the physical level. As a general rule a 6C should be used to start with when the emphasis of the symptoms lies mostly on the physical level and a 30C to start with when the emphasis is mainly emotional; such as the patient being extremely

angry, irritable or weepy, or if a baby is yelling its head off or a child stomping out of the room in a fury. If there are many emotional or mental symptoms and/or a great deal of energy shown by the patient then the potency to choose to start with should be a 200. I have mentioned when you should go straight to a 30C or higher in specific places in this book and occasionally I have referred to the 12C potency when it is a good potency to start with in those particular situations.

CHOOSING A POTENCY

Unless I have stated otherwise in the various chapters for particular ailments in this book always start by using the remedy in a 6C. If you find that the 6C seems to become less effective (but you are certain you still need that same remedy), you can start plussing it. To do this put about five pills (or five drops if you have a liquid remedy) into a glass of water and let them dissolve. (Some pills and tablets are slow to dissolve; if this is the case it is OK to crush them between two *clean* teaspoons first.) A dose then becomes a dessertspoonful of the liquid, to be held in the mouth for about half a minute or so in the usual way. However, *before* each time you take a dose you must (a) add a dessertspoonful of water to your glass to replace the water you removed for the previous dose and (b) stir the mixture thoroughly. By doing this you are diluting and giving (very mild) succussion to the remedy so that each dose becomes just a fraction higher in potency than before; this is very effective when the original potency seems to have 'run out of steam' and quite often makes it unnecessary to go up in potency to a 30.

For those of you who cannot be bothered with any plussing it would probably be advisable to have your most frequently required remedies in a 12C potency as well, so that you can use them if the 6C seems to become less effective. Obviously a 12C lies between a 6C and a 30C in energy. Many people prefer to go up from a 6C to a 12C rather than going directly up to a 30C when treating a patient, particularly if they do not want to do any plussing; also by going up to a 12C first, very often the 30C will not be required.

If you need to, you can either go straight up to a 30C after taking a 6C, or else you can plus the 6C and/or go up to a 12C first. Going up to a 200C would be the next potency after a 30C, or plussing a 30C. I have been deliberately vague here about how often you repeat a remedy, or how long you remain on a potency, because everyone's response is different and you must follow the advice in 'Rules about repetition of doses' below. All this may seem quite complicated but when you have done it once you will realize that it is really quite simple. *Never go back down in potency in the same remedy in the same acute illness.* In other words, do not go down from a 200C to a 30C or from 30C plussed to a 30C, or from a 30C to a 6C, or from 6C plussed to a 6C. It is perfectly OK, however, to go down in potency if you have changed the remedy. For example, if you had been giving Belladonna 30C you must not then go down to Belladonna 6C but you could give Bryonia 6C if the picture had changed and Bryonia was then indicated.

Also never go up to a 30, or start with a 30, just because you happen to think the disease is 'serious' and therefore needs a 'stronger' dose. This would only be reflecting *your* feelings and fears and would not be prescribing according to *how the patient actually is.* I have often found lay prescribers make this mistake. Many very serious complaints are cured completely by using 6C potencies; if you give the correct remedy but the potency is too high it may well not be very effective. Always follow the rules above and you will not go wrong.

Occasionally it is better to do the plussing in a bottle rather than in a glass. This is when the plussing procedure is likely to be continued over more than 36 hours or so and would usually be done under the supervision of a professional homoeopath. A 100 millilitre brown glass bottle is a good size for this; add a teaspoon of brandy or vodka to act as a preservative for the remedy and the water. Do not completely fill the bottle; up to about one inch or 2.5 centimetres from the top is about right. Otherwise you do it in exactly the same way as with the glass (in that you add a dessertspoonful of water each time to replace the previous dose), but the succussion is done by hitting the base of the bottle firmly into the palm of your hand twelve times before each dose.

The advantage of this method is that the succussion can be done *much* more efficiently and the remedy keeps better. It is unlikely that you would need to use this method for the types of ailments described in this book, but some people prefer doing it this way rather than in a glass (probably because the succussion process is more efficient), even if it is only for a short time or only for a few doses. Plussing is also extremely useful when you might be running out of a remedy, as it enables a very few pills to go further, lasting much longer.

DOSAGE

It is the **frequency of prescribing** the dose, **not the quantity of the remedy** which is important. In potencies from about a 6C upwards, it does not make any difference if you give one pill at a time or a bottle full, it has the same effect. This is because you are prescribing an energy not a measurable material quantity. So do not waste pills or drops by giving more on the assumption that if one pill helps, then more pills at a time will be even better. The frequency of prescribing must always be based on the advice in 'Rules about repetition of doses'.

RULES ABOUT REPETITION OF DOSES

The first and most important rule of all is: **As long as there is improvement in the patient do not repeat the remedy.** This is very important. Never give an extra dose 'just for luck'; quite apart from anything else it is a waste of medication and it can sometimes undo some of the good that has been achieved. You only repeat a remedy when the improvement seems to stop. It may help to bear in mind that **the remedy acts simply as a stimulus to the natural healing process of the body so that as soon as improvement begins you stop giving the remedy and let the body continue the healing process**.

Signs of improvement in acute situations:

a. The patient falls into a *peaceful* sleep.

b. The patient appears and feels a lot better.

c. The patient appears and feels a lot better in himself so that there is no suffering, or hardly any suffering, even though some or all of the physical symptoms are still there; physical improvement will follow shortly.

d. The patient vomits.

If any of the above happens after giving a remedy you can be sure that you prescribed the correct remedy and that cure has begun. Simply wait and watch and only represcribe when:-

a. Symptoms return.

b. The patient begins to feel the pain or discomfort again.

c. The improvement seems to reach a plateau, i.e. they are a bit better but progress seems to have come to a halt.

If you interfere too soon the progress that has been achieved could be arrested. Should you need to represcribe, make sure that the picture is still the same. If it has changed another remedy would be indicated.

If, however, the symptoms get worse, or the behaviour, gestures and actions of the patient indicate increased discomfort, then you have not given the remedy which is homoeopathic to the case and must reconsider before represcribing. The incorrect remedy itself will do no harm, in fact it will do absolutely nothing. However, such a mistake is a waste of time and prolongs the suffering of the patient.

It must be obvious from the above information that the frequency of prescribing varies from person to person according to the symptoms and their response to the remedy. Bear in mind that if someone has a high fever and/or is being 'energetically' ill, that is by being very restless or very emotional, they will appear to 'use up' the remedy faster and repetition will be more frequent. You might give one dose only and find that that is all that is required, or you may give a dose quite frequently, say about three times in the first hour, and then not need to give any more. You could find that you give a dose quite frequently for a few doses and then only need to give another dose or two quite a number of hours (or even a day or two) later, or you may find that the dose is required rather regularly every few hours for a day or more. *One mistake which people often make happens when any improvement lasts only for a very few minutes. I find that people either hardly notice the brief improvement, or consider that being so brief, it means that the remedy is not working. Such situations call for more patience and better observation. If the remedy has worked, even just for a few minutes, repeat it more often (i.e. whenever the symptoms relapse, which may be every few minutes) until improvement does last longer. If despite doing this, improvement does not begin to set in for any decent length of time, you should either start plussing the remedy or go up to the next potency.* If you follow the rules about prescribing given earlier in the section you will not go wrong. In all acute conditions the response to the remedy should be fairly immediate.

11. Introduction to using homoeopathy for first aid and acute diseases

When I refer to a 'dose', I mean one pill, or 2-3 drops of a liquid potency in about a teaspoonful of water, or a mouthful or dessert-spoonful if it is a remedy which has been plussed. As already mentioned it is a good idea to have certain remedies in liquid form, or as soft tablets, for babies and the very weak, as these are easier for them to take; but if you only have pills or tablets you can crush two or three between a couple of teaspoons and give the resulting powder; this is easier than trying to give them a pill. It makes no difference how many pills you use to crush up - remember you are giving an energy medicine which acts as a stimulus to the body's own healing powers; it is the frequency of the dose rather than the quantity which matters. I think it is always a good idea to have Arnica in a liquid potency as it is the remedy most frequently used if someone is unconscious or semi-conscious. Another remedy to have as a liquid potency might be Chamomilla; this is most frequently prescribed for babies when teething and it is much easier to give as a liquid than as crushed-up pills.

One of the most common pitfalls when prescribing for your family is that, because you are prescribing for those you care about most, it is very easy for your emotions to get in the way and affect the way you prescribe. When this happens you are likely to make mistakes. For this reason I have not only tried to make the advice as concise and clear as possible but have aimed at detachment, in the hopes that this will encourage you to be as detached as you can be when choosing a remedy. One helpful way to do this is to try to imagine yourself as the homoeopathic practitioner rather than the worried or possibly frightened person that you actually are. One mistake frequently made is that lay prescribers go up in potency too soon, often quite unnecessarily, reflecting *their own personal worries and anxieties* rather than following the rules and prescribing according to *how the patient actually is.* A second common mistake is that through impatience as well as anxiety lay prescribers do not calmly observe and take note of all the details of the symptoms; this is how important things get missed, an inaccurate picture is presented, and the wrong remedy chosen. The section on how to choose a remedy in an acute case (pages 25–26) should help. A third mistake which also tends to happen is that the remedy is changed too soon (or occasionally not soon enough), often through lack of observation or because the prescriber has forgotten about the 'signs of improvement' which should also be their guide and are described on pages 33–35. So be calm, be observant, try to be detached and remember to take your time choosing the remedy. If you get in a muddle go back to the basic rules on prescribing.

It is always a good idea to keep a record for each member of your family of what remedy you have prescribed and when, for what ailment and symptoms, as well as how effective it was and how quickly there was improvement. You will find this a great help when prescribing another time as many people often require the same remedy, or sequence of remedies, for particular types of illness. It will also save you a lot of time and will help you have a better under-standing of homoeopathy.

You will find other homoeopathic books with many more remedies in them which are just as effective, but in this book I have tried to stick to straightforward advice and to using only a small selection of the most frequently used remedies. In other books you will also find advice on how to treat many other more serious diseases. I do not think it a good idea for the layperson to treat diseases other than simple acute cases, accidents and injuries, because the only way to treat chronic diseases successfully is to have had a proper professional training; without this, serious conditions may be missed, underlying miasms ignored and the choice and knowledge of remedies would be extremely limited so that treatment will probably fail; the patient will be disappointed and might well end up discarding homoeopathy. Do-it-yourself homoeopathy is fine for the layperson to practise in acute cases providing they know what they are doing; it is definitely not a good idea for chronic diseases and you should study section 3, 'The difference between Acute and Chronic Conditions' to get a broader understanding of the subject.

If people are having any acute ailments very frequently, rather than just occasionally, it is very important that they consult a professional homoeopath in order to have treatment for the chronic underlying condition. In this way the tendency to develop such frequent acute conditions will be reduced and more serious disease will be prevented.

Chapter Two

ACCIDENTS, INJURIES
AND FIRST AID

This chapter covers the use of homoeopathy for treating accidents and injuries. It is essential that you have read and understood the whole of chapter one before you start using any homoeopathic remedies. This is so that you avoid making any mistakes in the choice of potency, repetition of a remedy or when handling the remedies. You will find that response to the homoeopathic remedy when treating accidents and injuries is remarkably fast and that consequently any suffering will be greatly reduced.

DOSAGE AND POTENCY GENERALLY

Throughout this chapter, unless I have indicated that you should use a specific potency for a particular situation or ailment, please remember to follow the advice given in the section on 'Rules about dosage, potencies and repetition of doses' on pages 30–35.

12. Emotional shock, trauma, fright, bad news

The following is for the *immediate* reactions to these traumas, not for any long-term suffering following an emotional trauma of any kind. For any long-term consequences, such as post-traumatic stress syndrome or grief, a professional homoeopath should be consulted as homoeopathy can dramatically help in preventing any serious disease and suffering, whether emotional or physical, resulting from the trauma. Those who need counselling or psychiatric help in these situations do extremely well when they combine this with homoeopathy; the therapies work very well together and I find that recovery is much quicker for those who have both rather than just the counselling on its own.

Arnica

This remedy is the main one for any kind of shock from an accident or injury; anything from the shock of a young child falling downstairs, to your family being involved in or witnessing a car accident. It is also useful for the shock resulting from receiving any seriously bad news. It is important to remember that what may not seem particularly traumatic to an adult may well be so to a child. The two main symptoms for Arnica are that the sufferers (1) insist they are perfectly well even if they are badly hurt and (2) do not want you to touch any physical injury or approach them in any way; this is easy to observe with children as they will scream out or make more fuss if they think you may be going to touch the injury. If they can they will move back from you if you get too close. They will seem dazed and may be incoherent. While some children may scream their heads off when in shock, others can remain unusually silent, so look out for this.

Rescue Remedy

This is one of the Bach remedies and is best used in liquid form, putting a few drops into a teaspoon of water and holding it in the mouth for up to about a minute before swallowing. Take two to three drops neat if water is unavailable. It does not come in a potency. Use it for any kind of shock or fright. It is a kind of alternative to Aconite and Arnica. Although improvement is usually fairly immediate this remedy needs to be taken regularly over a longer length of time than homoeopathic remedies. Perhaps half-hourly or more frequent doses during the initial shock or fright and then three to four times a day for a few days until the patient feels better.

Aconite

This is for shock combined with extreme fright. Those suffering will be very restless, frightened and are convinced they will die; older children and adults may even predict the time of death. It is quite often needed after the administration of Arnica because once the worst of any shock is over some fright may well remain from the trauma.

Ignatia

This remedy is chiefly for the immediate shock of grief or great loss. It is more often indicated for adults and older children and is particularly useful for the grief after someone has died as well as for grief following severe financial disaster or great disappointment. It is very useful for those experiencing redundancy, loss of promotion, great disappointments such as not being chosen for a much coveted position in a sports team, or being dropped from a team which they have been very proud to be in. It is also a remedy which is very helpful for anyone who may be hysterical with grief following the death of, or some kind of disaster to, someone in their family, a friend, a much admired hero, pop star or a much loved family pet. Mentally there will at the very least be a lot of sighing (although they may well not be aware of this); there will be restlessness, an inability to settle or get down to anything, and all the various degrees of misery as these emotional feelings build up to hysteria, as well as the hysteria itself. It is excellent to take before going to a funeral as well as at the time you first hear about a death. It is not usually a remedy for babies but even quite young children may require it if it fits their behaviour pattern and the situation.

DOSAGE AND POTENCY

The remedies used for these reasons are solely concerned with emotional symptoms so the potency used should be a 30, or a 30 plussed; occasionally you may need to go up to a 200 if the lower potency appears to have 'run out of steam'. The remedies should not be taken over more than about two to three days and usually only a few doses initially are required, with perhaps another dose occasionally if the symptoms return. (As you see, Rescue Remedy has a different dosage.)

13. Bruising and contused wounds, sprains and strains

A contusion is the same as a bruise, where the injury has pain, swelling and discolouration without the skin actually being broken. It usually results from impact against a hard, blunt object and is common in most accidents, many sports injuries as well as the kind of injuries children have around the house from falls, or from playing around with their brothers and sisters.

Arnica

This is the first and most important remedy to give. It deals with the shock as well as the bruising. However severe, deep or extensive the bruising, Arnica will help. The Arnica remedy picture is worse for touch and pressure; the pains are as if beaten, torn apart, or bruised. Mentally sufferers are better alone, they fear approach and touch and will insist that there is nothing wrong with them.

Dosage. You should give Arnica 30 or 200 if there are signs of *severe* shock when there are a lot of emotional symptoms, such as appearing dazed, bewildered and/or insisting they are feeling fine when they quite obviously are not; otherwise you should always start with Arnica 6. You may need to give this remedy quite often initially, such as every five to twenty minutes or so, but very soon the swelling and bruising will start to get better quite quickly and you will only need to repeat the remedy when the improvement slows down or stops.

Dressings. If necessary an Arnica lotion can be made up with one teaspoon Arnica Ø to one pint of water and applied with a dressing, but **Arnica lotion or Arnica Ø should never be applied to broken skin, nor should Arnica cream.** This is because some skins are sensitive to Arnica and it can produce a tiresome rash but only if the skin is broken.

Ledum

If any discolouration remains some time after administering Arnica and/or if the injury remains slightly swollen, Ledum will remove the discolouration and complete the healing. There will be the Ledum remedy picture of worse for warmth and touch, better for cold and uncovering.

Ruta

This is the remedy for (1) bruised, wrenched or torn tendons (a tendon is the same as a sinew and is the fibrous connective tissue which attaches muscles to bones), and (2) for kicks and knocks to the periosteum which is the fibrous membrane covering bones; it is for injuries to the parts where flesh is thin on the bones. A large number of sports injuries fit these two descriptions. I frequently need to give Ruta (following Arnica) to people who have been knocked or kicked during a game of football, cricket, or hockey. Bruising and kicks to shin bones; strained tendons; bruising from ill-fitting ski boots, and pain following osteopathic treatments are all types of injuries helped by Ruta. (Very occasionally Ruta does not completely cure periosteum injuries; if this is the case Symphytum should complete the cure.)

The Ruta remedy picture is worse for cold and better for warmth; worse for damp and wet weather; worse for exertion and better for gentle rubbing. The pains feel sore, lame and bruised. Nodes, nodules and bursae are helped by Ruta as well as injuries from overuse of a part of the body, such as a ganglion, tennis elbow, housemaid's knee and also some repetitive strain injuries; however a professional homoeopath should be consulted if these do not get better because sometimes they may be part of a much wider picture requiring constitutional treatment.

Symphytum

This remedy is a specific for bruising injuries to the eyeball, cheek bones and bones surrounding the eye. Injuries to these areas are particularly common in hockey games and car accidents; also when there are too many children in the back of a car and they do not all wear seat belts so that a child falls injuring this particular area of the face, or when the driver's head hits the steering wheel, the rest of the body being held back by the seat belt. Do not forget to give Arnica first for any shock and general bruising. This remedy is also very helpful for pain in the stump after the loss of a limb, see Hypericum below.

Rhus Tox.

This remedy is (1) for overstrain of muscles, stiffness from unusual overexertion and (2) for torn ligaments and tendons around joints, or sprains. Rhus Tox. is worse for the initial movement, better for continued movement and worse from overexertion. This can mean the stiffness on first rising from a chair or when getting out of bed in the morning, which eases off with movement but then comes back in time from overuse and tiredness. Rhus Tox. is worse for wet and damp weather and better for warmth and heat; better for rubbing and pressure. The pains are tearing, sore and bruised. I find this remedy very useful for those who are extremely competitive and consequently overexert themselves during sports and games, so that they get these kinds of aches and pains with the Rhus Tox. modalities. Rhus Tox. symptoms can also develop if, when hot and sweaty from exertion, people then sit around getting chilled without changing into dry clothes.

Hypericum

This is the remedy for any injuries to parts rich in nerves, such as shutting your fingers in a door, also for injuries to the spinal cord. It will also deal with any possibility of sepsis if the skin is actually broken (see sections 15, 16 and 17). Give Arnica first if the shock is bad. This remedy is also one of the remedies which are very useful for the phantom pain which can follow the loss of a limb; this pain is often excruciating and here you usually need Hypericum 200 or higher.

DOSAGE GENERALLY

For most injuries described above you will want to give Arnica first for the initial shock and bruising then follow it if necessary with whichever of the other remedies is most indicated. If shock is severe you may need to repeat the Arnica 30 a few times in the first hour but then spread it out with much longer intervals between doses, remembering only to repeat the dose if the symptoms return. The remedy you are giving for the physical injury may only be required three to four times a day for anything from about one day to a week; but again remember that the frequency varies for everyone and you must follow the 'Rules about dosage, potencies and repetition of doses' in section 10. Unless I have stated otherwise, always start with a 6C. I think you will be very surprised at how quickly your family gets better from these kinds of injuries.

14. Cuts (incised wounds) and abrasions, scratches and grazes

Cleaning Wounds

Clean the wound with water with a few drops of Calendula Ø in it, or use a Calendula lotion, (see Dressings/Lotions below). Calendula Ø acts as a kind of antiseptic. A little bleeding to help cleanse the wound should be allowed. Do not forget to give Arnica at this stage if there is any shock or bruising as well.

Haemorrhage

Firm pressure and raising the limb will stop most bleeding. You should apply Calendula Ø *undiluted* as it will dramatically help stop any bleeding. If a dressing is required always use a dry one, or one soaked in *neat* Calendula Ø if you are using Calendula Ø to stop any bleeding. (Only use a ligature if there is uncontrollable spurting bleeding and then remember to release the pressure about every fifteen to twenty minutes so that normal blood supply still reaches the limb, as without this gangrene can set in. A ligature should always be applied over a soft pad of some sort and not directly to the skin.) Calendula Ø is also very useful if there is a lot of bleeding after a tooth extraction.

DRESSINGS/LOTIONS

If bleeding is not much of a problem or once the bleeding is over and the wound cleaned up, and if you think a dressing is required, use a gauze dressing soaked and wrung out in Calendula or Hypericum lotion. This lotion should be made up with half a teaspoon of the Ø to half a pint of water. Dressings should be left undisturbed but can be kept damp with whichever lotion you are using. If the wound is extensive or deep give Calendula 6 or Hypericum 6 internally three times a day until it is clear that clean healing has set in. Later on Calendula or Hypericum cream will be preferred to a dressing.

Calendula or Hypericum

Use Hypericum 6 internally as well as Hypericum Ø externally for injuries which are (1) deep or extensive, (2) to areas rich in nerves (which are extremely painful), such as crushing one's fingers in the door, and (3) if there is any danger of tetanus (see section 15).

Use Calendula Ø (1) undiluted to stop any bleeding, and (2) as a lotion for cleaning up injuries.

Either Calendula or Hypericum can be used as a lotion for a dressing and/or internally in a 6C to promote clean healing and prevent sepsis. They are more effective if alternated rather than taken together in the form of Hypercal, although this is readily available in chemists and health food shops. Once healing has begun with whichever remedy you are using it is then best to alternate the Hypericum with the Calendula. You will probably want to switch to Hypericum or Calendula cream rather than using a lotion later on.

Children often get minor scratches and grazes from falling off their bicycles and playing about. Once they are cleaned up, Calendula or Hypericum cream is probably all that is required. The creams are available from health food shops as well as homoeopathic pharmacies. Adults will find both of them to be very good healing creams for scratched hands after gardening and any other scratches and grazes.

Staphisagria

This remedy is useful for really deep incisions and for incisions from surgery. Give Staphisagria 30 twice a day for a day or two if there is pain in the cut.

15. Punctured wounds

These wounds can be caused by any sharp pointed things such as sticking the prongs of a garden fork into one's foot, needle pricks and knife wounds. Treading on rusty nails or drawing pins is also a frequent cause of punctured wounds in children. The danger of these deeper injuries is the tetanus bacillus which can live in the soil and can grow anaerobically at the site of the injury. This means that it can only multiply in the absence of oxygen so the risk is much higher in deep punctured wounds than in grazes. Preventing tetanus with homoeopathic treatment is not complicated *providing treatment is started as soon as possible* after the injury. If you follow the advice in this section you should find that the improvement is remarkably fast.

CLEANING PUNCTURED WOUNDS; DRESSINGS

Wounds can be cleaned with water with a few drops of Calendula Ø in it. Hypericum Ø can then be put directly onto the wound or, if a dressing is required, make up a Hypericum lotion with one part Hypericum Ø to ten parts water and soak the dressing in this. With this and the appropriate internal remedy, the wound should heal up quickly and without infection.

Arnica

Give this first in a 30 for the shock, you may need to go up to a 200.

Ledum

The Ledum remedy picture is that of the punctured wound with shooting and pricking pains; puffy or dropsical swelling; the injured parts may feel cold to the touch although they may feel hot, not cold, to the sufferer. The wound is better for cold bathing, particularly in icy water, better for cold dressings, better for uncovering or exposure to cold air, worse for warmth and worse for any touch. If this remedy is indicated you may find the patient sitting with the injured hand, foot or whatever part of the body in a basin or bath containing icy cold water. You should alternate this remedy with Hypericum if there is any danger of tetanus. I often find it necessary to go up to a 30 with this type of injury.

Hypericum

This remedy is useful when the pain and/or red streaks from the punctured wound start to travel up the limb and the wound is very sensitive to touch; it is more tender than one would expect from the appearance of the wound. It is aggravated by cold and worse for motion. This remedy is often required following Ledum and is particularly indicated for injuries to areas rich in nerves. If there are any signs of the wound not healing cleanly alternate this remedy with Ledum and tetanus should be avoided. Start with Hypericum 6 but go up to a 30 and possibly a 200 later on if necessary.

Tetanus

The onset of tetanus is usually gradual although occasionally it may begin suddenly. First indications are stiffness of the jaw and neck muscles. In addition to the use of Hypericum alternated with Ledum as described earlier in this section, you could also use Tetanus 30 if you felt there was a real risk of the disease after an injury. For this give a dose of Tetanus 30 in the morning and evening of one day, and repeat a week later if necessary. An alternative way of prescribing is to give one dose of Tetanus 30 in the morning and evening of one day, then repeat every fourth day for three more doses. However the Ledum alternated with Hypericum is very effective.

The tetanus vaccine is now thought to have been purified so much, in order to make it safer, that its ability to prevent tetanus has been greatly reduced. Despite this, side effects from the vaccine can still cause fevers, nerve damage to the inner ear, degeneration of the nervous system and anaphylactic shock amongst other things. Also the vaccine has a preservative in it which contains mercury that, quite apart from anything else, is now thought to be extremely damaging to gums and to be a contributing factor in senile dementia.

16. Splinters and foreign bodies

Silica

You need to give this remedy first of all in order to push out any foreign body, such as a splinter or a thorn. In fact if there is the slightest difficulty getting the splinter out manually it is better to use Silica as it works so quickly and will be much less painful. Start with Silica 30, up to three doses daily for a few days; you will probably find only one or two doses will be necessary though, as the splinter will come out of its own accord very easily. This remedy will push out *any* foreign body (see warning note below) and will also help the body re-absorb or push out any pus round the injury if it has gone septic. It may well be the only remedy you require to heal up the injury.

Important note: Make sure you never give this remedy to anyone who has had a transplant of any kind, or a pacemaker, or has shrapnel from old war wounds or other injuries, as it is just possible that Silica could try to push these out too.

CLEANING SPLINTER-TYPE WOUNDS

Once you have removed the splinter, either manually or by giving Silica, wounds can be cleaned with water with a few drops of Calendula Ø in it. Hypericum Ø can then be put directly onto the injury, or if a dressing is required make up a Hypericum lotion with one part Hypericum Ø to ten parts water and soak the dressing in this; however, for these injuries which are usually quite small, a dressing is seldom needed.

Hepar Sulph.

Once the Silica 30 has pushed out the splinter, and only if the Silica does not appear to be helping get rid of the pus and heal the wound up (which it usually will do very efficiently), Hepar Sulph. 30 is a good alternative remedy. Use this remedy if the area round the wound is extremely painful, throbbing with pricking or sticking pains and very sensitive to touch (Silica is not worse for touch particularly, whereas Hepar Sulph. is). Hepar Sulph. is also worse for cold and worse for air; it is hot, highly inflamed, swollen and smelly, as well as having some pus. Only a few doses will be required. Generally speaking Hepar Sulph. should be used before Silica when there is pus as it is more useful in the earlier stages of an infected wound, but Silica would be used first when there is the necessity to push out a foreign body or splinter.

Belladonna

If the area round the wound is swollen, red, throbbing and hot but without there being any pus, take Belladonna 6 three to six times a day until it is better (but only after the Silica has pushed out the splinter). Probably only a very few doses will be required. I find this remedy the one most frequently used after getting thorns in one's fingers when gardening; once you have removed the thorn either manually or with Silica, it is the Belladonna picture of heat, throbbing, red, shiny swelling, worse for touch and cold, with no pus, that usually remains.

Hypericum

This remedy is useful when the pain and/or red streaks from the injury start to travel up the limb and the wound is very sensitive to touch; it is more tender than one would expect from the appearance of the wound.

Again you should use Silica first if the splinter is reluctant to come out. The wound is worse for cold and worse for motion. This remedy is often required following Ledum and is particularly indicated when the injury is to areas rich in nerves, such as one's fingertips. If there are any signs of the wound not healing cleanly, alternate this remedy with Ledum and tetanus should be avoided.

Ledum

Ledum is indicated if there are shooting and pricking pains in the area of the splinter and puffy or dropsical swelling. The parts feel cold to the touch (opposite to Belladonna) although they may feel hot, not cold, to the sufferer. The wound is better for cold bathing, even better for icy cold water, better for cold dressings, better for cold air and uncovering, worse for warmth and worse for any touch. You must not forget to use Silica first if the splinter will not come out on its own. You should alternate this remedy with Hypericum if there is any danger of tetanus.

Tetanus

In addition to the use of Hypericum alternated with Ledum as described earlier in this section you could also take Tetanus 30 if you felt there was a risk of the disease after an injury. For this give a dose in the morning and evening of one day and repeat a week later if necessary; or else one dose in the morning and evening of one day and then one dose every fourth day for three more doses. On the whole this remedy should not really be needed if you use the Ledum alternated with Hypericum as necessary (see section 15 on tetanus).

Aconite

I find this remedy very useful for eyes that are inflamed as a result of having had a foreign body in them. The eye feels dry, burning, as if full of sand and is worse for light. These symptoms can also come on from exposure to cold, dry, windy weather. It is also very good in helping with the fright and panic people often experience with any sort of eye injury.

Euphrasia

This is a remedy which is excellent for eye injuries. Take Euphrasia 6 internally as required. You can also use this remedy to bathe the eye to remove any foreign body from it, and to soothe the eye afterwards. Put two to three drops *only* of Euphrasia Ø into an eyebath of boiled then cooled water and bathe your eye with this. It is very refreshing and cooling for tired eyes, and is particularly helpful for contact lense wearers for bathing the eyes.

17. Lacerated wounds

These wounds involve bruising and damage to tissues as well as broken skin. First of all you should give Arnica for the shock, then clean the wounds with water with a few drops of Calendula Ø in it. Continue with Arnica while you decide whether or not a more appropriate remedy for the injury should be given. For this look up the remedies for 'Bruising and contused wounds', 'Cuts (incised wounds) and abrasions', 'Punctured wounds' and 'Broken and cracked bones' in sections 13, 14, 15 and 20. The summary below should help you decide. These types of injuries can occur playing sports but are also caused by falls from trees or climbing frames, the elderly falling over or tripping up, or as a result of do-it-yourself, road and other accidents.

Antiseptic:	Calendula or Hypericum internally and externally (alternated)
Broken bones:	Symphytum (Arnica, Hypericum initially)
Bruising:	Arnica, Hypericum, Ruta, Symphytum, Rhus Tox., Ledum
Cheek bones:	Symphytum (Arnica initially)
Cuts:	Staphisagria, Hypericum, Calendula

Eyeball injury:	Symphytum (Arnica initially)
Eye:	Symphytum, Aconite, Euphrasia
Haemorrhage:	Calendula Ø externally neat (or on dry dressing), Arnica internally
Kicks and knocks:	Ruta (Arnica initially)
Limb, pain moving up from injury:	Hypericum (alternate with Ledum and/or Tetanus)
Nerves, damage to:	Hypericum (may need Arnica initially)
Periosteum damage:	Ruta (parts where flesh is thin on bones), Symphytum, (Arnica initially)
Punctured wounds:	Ledum, Hypericum, Tetanus, Belladonna (Arnica initially)
Scratches/abrasions:	Calendula, Hypericum
Splinters/thorns:	Silica, Hepar Sulph., Belladonna, Ledum, Hypericum, Tetanus, Aconite
Sprains:	Rhus Tox. (Arnica initially)
Stiff muscles:	Rhus Tox.
Strained muscles:	Rhus Tox.
Tendons, damage to:	Ruta (Arnica initially)
Tetanus (preventative):	Ledum alternated with Hypericum, Hypericum dressings, Tetanus 30.

More often than not you will be surprised at the speed of recovery but very occasionally pain, discomfort or weakness may persist to some extent despite giving the remedies. In these cases consult a professional homoeopath as a deeper acting or constitutional remedy may be required to complete the job.

18. Bites and stings

Ledum

Ledum is the main remedy for most bites, stings and punctured wounds. Use it for dog bites, wasp stings, bee stings and mosquito bites. If the bites are not particularly severe or extensive start with Ledum 6 and plus it if necessary. For deeper, more severe or more numerous bites use Ledum 30, but you may need to go up to 200. Some children can be vulnerable to getting bitten by dogs as they tend to tease a dog, which though generally friendly and safe, then gets overexcited or angry. Ledum would be very helpful for treating such bites and the injury will heal up very quickly.

The Ledum remedy picture is that of the punctured wound or sting with shooting and pricking pains; puffy or dropsical swelling; the parts feel cold to the touch although they may feel hot not cold to the sufferer. They are relieved by cold bathing, even more so in icy cold water, better for cold air and for uncovering, worse for warmth, and worse for any touch.

Apis

Apis is particularly useful for bee stings. If anyone in your family keeps bees Apis 6 should be taken just before doing anything with their hive, and any stings will hardly be felt. The Apis remedy picture has a lot of burning and stinging pains as well as the rapid swelling of the injured part. Apis is worse for heat and hot applications, better for cool air and cold applications. There may be trouble urinating, (frequency or retention) which can happen if there have been many stings. Use Apis 6 plussing it if necessary or go straight up to Apis 30. Apis is also very good for jellyfish stings (as is Medusa) so take it with you when you go to the seaside.

Hypericum

This remedy is very useful when the pain shoots up the nerve of the limb from the bite or sting. The wound is worse for cold and very sensitive to the touch. Start with Hypericum 30.

Belladonna

Very occasionally this remedy is required when some of the modalities are opposite to those of Apis and Ledum; that is if the wound is hot (Ledum is actually cold, although to the patient it feels hot) and is worse for cold. The area round the wound is swollen, red, throbbing and hot but without having any pus.

Vipera

Use this remedy as a specific against the British adder. If you do not have it with you choose the most similar remedy going by the presenting symptoms. Vipera is best used in a 30C.

Carbolicum Acidum

This remedy is most useful after very extensive wasp or bee stings when the sufferer has possibly encountered a swarm, or else when one or more stings are in very sensitive areas such as inside or very close to the mouth, lips, eyes, ears or nose. Unfortunately, if young children are frightened of wasps or bees they tend to hit out at them which makes the insects angry; the children then scream with their mouths wide open - making themselves very vulnerable to being stung in one of the most sensitive places. Carbolicum Acidum is also useful for adder bites and other snake bites. With this remedy picture the sufferer appears extremely lethargic or prostrated or perhaps may even be losing consciousness. The pulse will be feeble and the breathing stertorous and laborious, and they will be bathed in cold sweat. The face will be very pale or dusky in appearance and there will be increased thirst. With this kind of situation the deterioration may well be fast and it is essential to give Carbolic. Acid. 30 as soon as possible, repeating it as necessary. Recovery should be fast.

Vespa Crabro

All wasp stings are unpleasant and painful, but some types of more aggressive wasps have very much fiercer stings; this remedy is preferable to Apis in such cases, as well as being very good for dealing with stings from hornets. A key indication for this remedy is the intense violent itching and prickling in the area of the sting, which usually extends well beyond just the sting area. In extreme cases there can also be breathing difficulties and drowsiness much like Carbolic. Acid. It is best to start with a 30.

DOSAGE

Initially you may need to give the remedy quite frequently following the bite or the sting, maybe three to six times during the first hour or two, (sometimes every few minutes initially); thereafter it will be required much less often and should only be given if and when the symptoms return. Always follow the advice in section 10 on 'Rules about dosage, potencies and repetition of doses'. I think you will be very surprised at how fast the recovery is. Do not forget to give Arnica 30 if there is shock or Aconite 30 if there is severe fright.

For severe poisonings, for example from snake bites, a ligature should be applied between the bite and the heart so as to prevent the poison circulating. Any ligature should be as tight as possible (although not directly onto the skin) and should leave some pulse below it. It should be relaxed every 15–20 minutes for about one minute. Poison can be sucked out of a wound providing there are no cracks or sore places on the lips or in the mouth. There are many other remedies for snake bites which are beyond the scope of this book, but if you and your family are travelling in areas where you are likely to encounter snakes, consult a homoeopath beforehand so as to be prepared with the appropriate remedies. If the snake venom is known you can give it in the 30th potency and for jellyfish stings you can use Medusa 30 or Apis.

CLEANING AND DRESSING DOG BITES AND SIMILAR WOUNDS

Wounds can be cleaned with water with a few drops of Calendula Ø in it. Hypericum Ø can then be put directly onto the bites, but if the bites are extensive and a dressing is required, make up a Hypericum lotion with one part Hypericum Ø to ten parts water and soak the dressing in this. With this and the appropriate internal remedy the wound should heal up quickly and without any sign of infection.

OTHER EXTERNAL APPLICATIONS AND PREVENTATIVES FOR BITES AND STINGS

Wine vinegar or cider vinegar, either neat or diluted, can be dabbed onto minor bites and stings. Alternatively Urtica Urens Ø or Ledum Ø can be used on wasp and bee stings, Calendula Ø or Hypericum Ø (or Hypercal) on mosquito and gnat bites, and Hypericum Ø for snake bites. There is a Pyrethrum spray which is very effective in preventing bites and stings from insects and it is also very good to dab Pyrethrum Ø on bites and stings; this immediately removes any itching and stinging, and brings great relief.

19. Burns

If you try to combine allopathic treatment or dressings with homoeopathic treatment for burns, the homoeopathic treatment may not work or at best may be very slow and there may be scarring. This is one instance where it is particularly important that you stick to one form of treatment or the other. You will find homoeopathy works very quickly. Using the appropriate homoeopathic treatment for burns makes the use of skin grafts virtually unnecessary, scarring is minimal (usually there is none at all), the injury heals extremely quickly and the suffering and pain are a great deal less. By using homoeopathy for these injuries you will save a great deal of time and suffering, when you might otherwise have been visiting the patient in hospital while skin grafts are done; you will also save the patient a lot of embarrassment, teasing, and sometimes unhappiness later on in life as most scarring, if not all scarring, should have been avoided as well as the grafts themselves.

It is important to be aware that most accidents which occur in the home occur in the kitchen, one of the most common being a child spilling boiling water from the kettle, usually over the arm and hand. This often happens when children are just old enough to try and be helpful and do things for themselves, but still too young to be fully aware of the danger.

FIRST DEGREE BURNS

Urtica Urens

First degree burns are superficial, and the damage is only to the outer layer of the skin with no blistering. Here use Urtica Urens both internally and externally. Give Urtica Urens 30 and it will relieve the pain in about seven minutes. Repeat the remedy whenever the pain returns. The remedy may be all you need, but if necessary make up a lotion of half a teaspoon of Urtica Urens Ø to half a pint of water and soak a pad of gauze in this for a dressing to cover the whole area of the burn. Whenever the dressing begins to dry, soak it with the lotion again. The dressing should not be disturbed once it has been applied. Later on you can use Urtica Urens cream, or Hypericum or Calendula cream, to complete the healing. Urtica Urens 30 is one remedy which it is useful to keep near the kitchen in case you burn yourself on a saucepan or oven door. Urtica Urens is also very good for sunburn when it fits the Urtica description; usually Urtica Urens 6 will be the potency required for this.

Vitamin E

An alternative to Urtica is to use vitamin E capsules. Simply snip the capsule open, squeeze the contents over the burn and keep the area covered with the vitamin E oil, making sure it does not dry up. Although this is only practical if the area is very small, it is very effective.

Both methods should heal the burn with no scarring in a remarkably short time. Taking vitamin E internally also helps prevent scarring.

SECOND AND THIRD DEGREE BURNS

Causticum

For burns to the limbs, when there is blistering (but no actual charring), pain and restlessness, and the tissue is still pink, not white or coagulated, the remedy to use is Causticum 30. The pain should go within 7–10 minutes and the remedy should be repeated whenever the pain returns. Make up a Hypericum lotion of one teaspoon Hypericum Ø to a pint of water, soak a gauze dressing in this and cover the whole area. Keep the dressing damp but do not disturb it once it has been applied. If there is no improvement in the pain within ten minutes, consider giving Cantharis if the symptoms fit that picture better.

Cantharis

This is indicated (a) for any second or third degree burn to the face, chest or abdomen, (b) if the burn is extensive, (c) if there is a lot of blistering, tissue is white, coagulated or charred and (d) if there is extreme shock. In any of these situations the remedy to use is Cantharis 30, if the burn is very severe or extensive start with a 200. The pain will disappear in less than ten minutes and the remedy should be repeated whenever the pain returns. A Hypericum dressing should be applied as described above and kept damp with the Hypericum lotion, taking care not to disturb the dressing. The Cantharis will also help the painful micturition which may follow a severe burn of this kind. I find I use this remedy more frequently than Causticum (see above). I think you will be amazed at the speed with which healing occurs and pain is relieved.

ADDITIONAL NOTES

Do not forget to give a dose of Arnica if there is shock or Aconite if there is severe fright. Always give the burn remedy first (Urtica, Causticum or Cantharis) so that the pain goes away then decide whether to give Arnica or Aconite from time to time if required. For severe burns I would start giving the Arnica or Aconite in a 200 if necessary. I find children in particular nearly always need Aconite at some stage when treating their burns.

Later on, when healing has begun, you can either apply Calendula cream to the edges of the burn and Hypericum cream to the rest of the burn, or else you can alternate between the two, changing them whenever the healing seems to slow down. Calendula and Hypericum work much better if they are alternated rather than given combined in the form of Hypercal.

There can be complications following third degree burns in which case other remedies may well be indicated. There is, however, absolutely no reason why you should not get started with the treatment outlined above immediately, as pain should cease and healing commence. If necessary you should follow this up with a visit to your homoeopath as soon as possible in the more severe cases.

20. Broken and cracked bones

Start by giving Arnica at once to prevent shock and to reduce swelling and bruising. Any swelling, puffiness and bruising will disappear very quickly so that the bones can be set. If there has been damage to the nerves, give Hypericum 6, repeating it whenever the pain returns. You should follow these with Symphytum 6 three times a day for two weeks; after five days off it, you can repeat it for two more weeks if necessary and you should find that the healing takes about half the usual time. It is important to start Symphytum only **after** the bones are set straight, as it speeds up the healing so much that the bones could start to heal up crooked, if taken too soon. I find that higher potencies are required if the break is either close to, or in, a joint. If there is still some residual bruising later on (sometimes even after the plaster has been removed), use Ledum 6 three times a day for a day or two until it has gone.

When the bones are just cracked or not put in a plaster, take Symphytum 6 three times a day for the first few days (after initial doses of Arnica and/or Hypericum) and then repeat only when any pain returns; it will speed up the healing and act as a marvellous painkiller. Constitutional homoeopathic treatment is needed for those rare occasions when a bone refuses to heal.

21. Surgery and operations

Any operation, even quite a minor one, is a shock to the system. Shock is one of the main causes of things going wrong during or after surgery. If surgery is required following an accident of some kind then it is even more important to eliminate shock as much as possible. Providing that you yourself are calm and not overanxious, it is best to stay with patients as long as possible before the operation and be with them as much as you can afterwards.

Arnica

Use this remedy to prevent any shock from surgery and to help with the subsequent bruising and pain. It also reduces bleeding which makes things much easier for the surgeon. If you give the patient a couple of drops of Arnica 30 as late as you are allowed to before the operation (it is best to have your Arnica 30 in a liquid potency for these occasions) and then at least three to four times a day for the next one to three days you will find recovery time much quicker than expected and the pain and bruising will be much less. Remember to stop the remedy as soon as there is improvement and restart if symptoms return. Do not forget to use it for dental surgery as well. Occasionally I have had patients whose surgeons, in ignorance, prescribed Arnica daily for a number of weeks before surgery. These patients then started proving the Arnica, (see page 4) becoming severely bruised and in a worse state than if nothing had been taken at all; so always consult a homoeopath about homoeopathic treatment, not an allopath!

Aconite

Sometimes there can be great restlessness, fear and/or anxiety a day or two before an operation. If this is the case a dose of Aconite 30 will help tremendously. This remedy is very helpful for those who find the strangeness of the hospital environment very frightening; some children can get very panicky when their parents leave.

Gelsemium

Occasionally you find there is actual shaking and trembling from fear at the thought of having an operation; a few doses of Gelsemium 30 are very calming.

Phosphorus

This is the main remedy which should be considered for those who are badly affected by anaesthetic. It is particularly indicated if they come out of the anaesthetic very slowly and if post-operative vomiting is prolonged. They desire cold drinks which they then vomit not long after drinking; they cannot keep anything down and may have burning pains in the stomach.

Rescue Remedy

Some people can become very distressed and scream and cry out after surgery while they are still unconscious. If you are able to be with them at this time you can put a couple of drops of Rescue Remedy or Arnica onto the tongue or lips every few minutes. They should calm down very quickly so that healing from the operation can begin. Only give them more if the symptoms return. If you yourself find this time very trying you should take Rescue Remedy yourself. This is one of the Bach remedies and works best taken as a liquid. It does not come in a potency.

Bellis Perennis

This is an excellent remedy to take for any major abdominal surgery.

Once you have given Arnica 30 for a day or two after the operation go on to Bellis Perennis 6, or 30 if necessary, three or more times a day for a few days; remembering to stop as soon as there is improvement. Bellis Perennis is particularly indicated for wounds and surgery to the abdominal, uterine and breast area. It should prevent bruising and sepsis to these areas, thus speeding up the healing process dramatically. You will find that the surgeon will be astonished at the speed of recovery. It also reduces pain and discomfort after a woman has had a contraceptive coil fitted or removed, or has had a smear test.

Staphisagria

This remedy is useful for really deep incisions such as the kind which occur from surgery. If there is any pain in the incision after all the bruising has gone (and Arnica or Bellis Perennis or any other remedy is no longer needed) then this is the time to give Staphisagria 30 twice a day for a day or two; only repeat the remedy if the pain returns. Staphisagria can also be taken in this way for pain in any surgical incision even if it is many years since the operation.

22. Childbirth: some first aid measures

There are a few first aid procedures you can use which will make labour much easier and less traumatic both for you and your baby. If you want more individual help from a homoeopath you will find that most homoeopaths are happy to assist at the birth. They will be able to choose from the vast number of remedies which may be required during labour to make the birth as straightforward and painless as possible; these remedies can help with many of the complications, however serious, which can sometimes occur. Homoeopathy used during pregnancy will help with other individual problems such as morning sickness, as well as after the birth if you are unlucky enough to develop post-natal depression or other conditions. Here it is best to consult your homoeopath.

Arnica

Arnica 30 should be used 2-4 hourly during labour to help prevent bruising and shock for the mother as well as the baby; shock is a major cause of things going wrong during labour, so if necessary go up to a 200. Arnica is particularly helpful during forceps deliveries as it will prevent the sometimes severe bruising to the baby's head as well as the shock from what is usually, by then, a prolonged delivery.

Clary Sage

This is an aromatherapy oil. Before you go into labour mix up a 30–50 ml size bottle of it. The quantities are three drops of Clary Sage oil per 5 ml teaspoon of carrier oil. Any vegetable oil (such as olive oil or sunflower oil) will serve as a carrier oil although some mothers prefer to use a carrier oil obtained from a health food shop. Make sure that the Clary Sage oil you buy has not already been diluted. Use this mixture to rub on both your abdomen and your back as frequently as required during labour. You will find it will dramatically reduce the abdominal pains and get rid of most of the backache. It should *not be used* for backache during pregnancy itself but it is excellent during labour. Keep this oil separate from your homoeopathic remedies as you do not want the smell to antidote the remedies by mistake.

Caulophyllum

This remedy is indicated very frequently when the mother feels shaky and tremulous *with* intermittent, irregular labour pains, which often fly around in all directions but never in the right direction. This picture may occur with (1) false labour pains, (2) labour pains ceasing from exhaustion, (3) pains which are weak and irregular or else very severe; whichever is the picture dilation is extremely slow, no progress seems to be being made and labour is prolonged. Any of this may sometimes be accompanied by quite severe painful swelling of the finger joints. (There are many other remedies for slow progress and slow dilation during childbirth but they are beyond the scope of this book. It depends so much on the individual picture presented by the mother at the time, which is why it is preferable to have a homoeopath present at the birth.) It is also useful when the baby is overdue. Take a 30, two to three times a day for up to a week, and hopefully you will not have to have the baby induced. Occasionally I have had patients who have had to go up to a 200 for this to be successful.

Chamomilla

This is particularly useful when labour pains begin in the back and travel down the inner thighs. Such pains may be accompanied by over-excitement, nervousness and very frequently by anger.

Rescue Remedy

Like all Bach remedies this does not come in a potency. Take two to three drops direct onto the tongue, or preferably in a teaspoonful of water, as often as you need it. It will help with shock, fear, panic, exhaustion and the pain in a very general way during labour. It is a remedy you could alternate with Arnica. Like Arnica it is useful in preventing shock in your newly born baby. Remember it is the frequency of the dose, not the quantity, which matters. Do not forget that your husband may need it as well!

Calendula

If you make up a Calendula lotion you can use it to heal an episiotomy or any tearing which may occur. The lotion should be made with one part Calendula to twenty parts water and it is a good idea to make it up before the birth; you then soak a dressing in the lotion and place it against the wound, keeping the dressing damp. You should find it heals up without any sepsis and about twice as fast as is normally expected.

CAESAREAN SECTION

If you find yourself needing a Caesarean section, whether planned or as an emergency during labour, use the remedies as indicated in section 21 on 'Surgery and operations'. Start off with Arnica and then go on to Bellis Perennis. You may well need Staphisagria later on. You will find you will heal up and feel better much faster than those around you who are not using homoeopathy.

Chapter Three

COMMON ACUTE AILMENTS

This chapter covers the acute illnesses which occur most frequently. It is very important to remember that acute ailments do not just happen out of the blue; they are always part of a much deeper chronic underlying condition. The healing energy which we all possess is always repairing and maintaining the body and does this by protecting the most important and innermost parts of us and pushing disease outwards. When our healing energy succeeds in doing this an acute illness of some kind will emerge. This is an excellent thing to happen and it is crucial that the symptoms are not suppressed and driven back inwards (as often happens with ordinary medicine), but are cured by a homoeopathic remedy going along with and encouraging the action of the natural healing energy in the body. If you are able to use homoeopathy to treat these acute diseases when they occur, you and your family should be much stronger and healthier after the illness than before, and the illness itself should be much less severe and of shorter duration.

23. Fevers

I am going to divide the fever remedies into fast onset remedies, when the symptoms develop over a matter of hours, and slow ones which develop over a number of days. Fevers may precede or accompany many different illnesses such as influenza and bad colds (which may lead to coughs and pneumonia), otitis media, teething, meningitis and the acute childhood diseases. On these occasions if you use homoeopathy, not only does the illness not last long, but also the consequent feelings of weakness and exhaustion, including any subsequent complications, should be prevented. Any more serious diseases should be nipped in the bud, or if they do develop they should be comparatively mild. Homoeopathic medicine has numerous remedies for fevers so I am going to give the most common ones for those fevers to which the British climate makes us more susceptible. Obviously fevers in countries with very different climates will require a different selection of main remedies.

DOSAGE AND POTENCIES

Throughout this chapter, unless I have indicated that you should use a specific potency for a specific situation or ailment, please remember to follow the advice given in the section on 'Rules about dosage, potencies and repetition of doses' on pages 30–35.

When treating people with fevers, it is important to remember that if the temperature is very high the remedy gets used up quite fast and may need to be repeated quite often, *but only whenever the symptoms return*. Do not forget that children tend to run much higher temperatures than adults. Do not mess up your homoeopathic treatment by suddenly prescribing calpol or paracetamol as this will alter and confuse the picture; you would then be more likely to choose the wrong remedy and delay cure. In this chapter the 'Causes' indicate whatever might have increased the susceptibility to becoming ill and developing fever symptoms. Start with a 30 if the Mentals are very prominent; often the only potency you will need will be a 6. Signs of improvement (see section 10) should follow in ten to twenty minutes (often within one minute or less). If improvement does not occur and you are *sure* of the remedy, repeat it more often or else go up in potency. You will usually find you will not have long to wait. If improvement lasts only a few minutes this does not necessarily mean it is the wrong remedy; it may simply need to be given more frequently or in a higher potency.

FAST ONSET FEVERS

Belladonna

Causes   Exposure to cold, wet weather (or very hot sun, see 'Sunstroke', section 31). Washing or cutting the hair, particularly if it is not dried immediately.

Fever The onset is fast and the sufferer is burning hot. The skin is red and dry, but is probably damp hot and sweaty under the hair and under the clothes or bedclothes; that is they are sweaty on the parts which are covered up. The pupils are dilated, eyes bloodshot and there may be lachrymation. Patients want the light off and the curtains drawn because their eyes are worse for light. They want the door and windows shut and the bedclothes drawn up as they are worse for draughts, and they may feel very cold in themselves even when feverish. They are angry, irritable and cross, rather than frightened; and at best are grumpy, difficult and fairly hard to please. They are hypersensitive to any noise as well as to light, draughts and cold. Symptoms are frequently very right sided. Patients are worse, or the symptoms come on initially, at around 3 am or 3 pm. They are thirsty, particularly for lemonade. If they can they prefer to be lying half propped against the pillows, particularly if they have a headache. Pains are throbbing or pulsating, cramping or spasmodic. There is a lot of restlessness and if the temperature goes really high there may be delirium, when they think they see monsters and so on, and they may become violent and throw themselves around.

Dosage Unless the patient is delirious or extremely angry and restless, start with Belladonna 6. Plus the Belladonna 6 if there comes a time when you feel it is becoming less effective, only going up to a 30 if necessary. If there is extreme restlessness and/or anger start with Belladonna 30 and plus it later on if necessary. If there is delirium start with Belladonna 200. Whatever the severity of the fever, some degree of improvement should happen within minutes of giving the dose. Repeat the remedy only when improvement lapses. This may be anything from a few minutes to a few hours.

Aconite

Causes Exposure to cold, dry weather, particularly if windy, or from frights.

Fever   There is a sudden onset of the fever. Aconite types are extremely restless, they throw off the bedclothes and feel better for uncovering. The face particularly and the skin generally are very red, hot, dry and burning. There is burning thirst. The pupils are contracted and the eyes worse for light. Patients are worse at about 9 pm until about midnight and sometimes at 9 am as well. Mentally they are extremely restless and fearful; often they think they are so ill they are about to die. When well the Aconite type is more likely to have ruddy cheeks and seem quite strong and healthy, quite different from the pale, easily tired Ferrum Phos. type (see below). The red face can go quite pale when they sit or stand up, and this symptom must not be confused with the alternation between flushing and growing pale of Ferrum Phos.

Dosage   If there is not too much restlessness and fear start with Aconite 6 and go up later on if necessary. If the main features are the restlessness and fear start with Aconite 30. As the patient improves after the administration of Aconite you will find him starting to sweat; this is not necessarily a contra-indication for Aconite (which is a very dry remedy) but the rest of the picture must still be Aconite if he is to have another dose. Aconite is usually only useful in the early stages of a fever. If there is extreme restlessness and fear go up to a 200.

Ferrum Phos.

Fever   Again this remedy is used in the first stages of fever and, like Aconite and Belladonna, this remedy will abort a feverish cold and/or flu if given in time and if the remedy picture fits the symptoms. The sufferer is not as 'energetically' sick as Aconite or Belladonna but equally is not as sluggish or as lethargic as Gelsemium (see the slow onset fevers). When compared to other remedies Ferrum Phos. may seem rather nondescript, and this can be a guiding symptom. By this I mean that as well as having the Ferrum Phos. symptoms there will not be very specific temperament, time, side, weather or temperature aggravations which would indicate any other remedy. Ferrum Phos. types tend to alternate between being either flushed or pale and if you are not very observant this very important symptom is easy to miss. They are generally better for air. Mentally they tend to be dissatisfied and indifferent rather than irritable, and occasionally may be excitable. They prefer to be left alone and not bothered. The onset is sudden, with local congestion and inflammation. It is particularly suitable for those who tend to be rather pale when well and are not very robust.

SLOW ONSET FEVERS

Gelsemium

Causes Warm, wet, humid weather, mild damp winters, and humid summers.

Fever This develops slowly over about two or three days. The head, eyelids and limbs feel very heavy. Sufferers are drowsy and lethargic, the eyelids appear to droop half open and their eyes ache particularly. They complain of great weight, tiredness and aching over the whole body with a lack of muscular co-ordination. They can have cold shivers which travel up and down the back even though they are generally hot and sticky. They are usually thirstless even though their mouth and lips are dry. They may be shaking or tremulous which is particularly noticeable if they are holding something, and they are very low in energy and weak. They want to lie half reclined and generally get relief from profuse urination particularly if they have a headache. They want to be alone, not wanting anyone there at all, even if the other person is completely silent; this is quite a surprising symptom in young children, so it is sure to catch your attention.

Dosage   Start with Gelsemium 6; with such low energy one seldom needs to go very high with this remedy.

Bryonia

Causes   Cold dry east winds, cold dry weather, hot weather, financial worries.

Fever   This is a slow onset remedy from exposure to cold, dry, windy weather (whereas Aconite is a fast onset remedy from cold, dry, windy weather). There is extreme thirst and the mouth, lips and surrounding area are dry and often red and sore. The tongue is dry too and the taste is bitter. The eyes can be sore and moving the eyeballs is uncomfortable. Generally patients are very much worse for movement and lie very still, but sometimes their aches and pains can make them restless which can be confusing. The main thing is that they are worse not better for movement. They are better for hard firm pressure although worse for light touch. They are worse for warmth and better for cool air. They can become delirious and then will talk about 'going home', even if they are already at home. Their mood is irritable and they definitely want to be left alone.

Dosage   Start with a 30 or 200 if they are already delirious, otherwise start with a 6.

Rhus Tox.

Causes   Exposure to cold, wet, damp weather. Getting cold when sweating, for instance after sports activities.

Fever   This is a slow onset fever from getting cold and wet, whereas Belladonna is a fast onset fever from cold and wet exposure. This remedy has severe aching in the limbs, stiffness and bruising pains. Rhus Tox. pains mostly affect the muscles whereas Eup. Perf. pains mostly affect the bones. The pains are worse for rest and worse for the initial movements, but better with continued motion; this leads to tremendous restlessness, tossing and turning. They may prefer to lie on something hard. They sweat quite a lot, feeling extremely hot inside but icy cold on the surface. They are worse for draughts and uncovering, and better for warm wraps, hot baths and rubbing. If you look at their tongue it probably has a bright red triangular area at the tip. Sometimes there can be some urticaria (itchy eruption often in wheals) accompanying the fever and this improves and disappears as the fever breaks and they start to sweat. Mentally, apart from their restlessness, they are very despairing and possibly weepy about their aches and pains. They are thirsty, particularly for milk.

Eupatorium Perfoliatum

Fever   This fever remedy can be confused with Rhus Tox. as Eup. Perf. also has the severe bruised, aching pains, but in fact these pains are much worse in the bones than those of Rhus Tox; it feels as if the bones are breaking and the pains are much more violent. Also the fever comes on slightly quicker than Rhus Tox. Unlike Rhus Tox., the sufferer dares not move for the pains although at times you find the pains drive them to restlessness (Bryonia). One unusual thing is that they are not particularly sweaty despite the fever. The eyeballs may feel sore like Bryonia and Gelsemium. They tend to be very thirsty for cold water and will vomit anything they eat or drink. It is a particularly useful remedy if the sufferer is already worn out for any reason such as from illness or age.

24. Colds and sore throats

If there is a tendency to get many colds each winter, or very severe colds, it is much better to get constitutional treatment for this from your homoeopath. This will improve the general health so that people are much less susceptible to succumbing to colds in the first place. You should also visit your homoeopath if unpleasant symptoms persist despite the acute homoeopathic remedy, because the following is a selection only of the most commonly used remedies for colds; there is always a chance that a less usual remedy will be needed. It is extremely important not to suppress a cold with allopathic medication (this tends at the very least to cause headaches and sinus problems) as the discharge is part of the body's efforts to throw off some of the toxic material we accumulate over the years. The homoeopathic remedy goes along in the same direction as this natural healing process, speeding it up, so that the cold will go much more quickly, and afterwards the patient should feel generally healthier than before. As far as feverish colds are concerned you should also read section 23 on 'Fevers' for the remedies Belladonna, Aconite, Ferrum Phos., Gelsemium, Bryonia and Rhus Tox. so as to get a full picture of the fevers for these remedies. When treating sore throats you can also look up 'Diphtheria' in section 42 for more extensive descriptions of the remedy pictures for throat symptoms. Do not forget that ordinary medicaments for colds and sore throats usually contain substances such as menthol or eucalyptus, which antidote homoeopathic remedies (see pages 23–25) and therefore must be avoided.

Aconite

Colds This remedy is for the *first sign* of a cold following exposure to cold, raw, dry, windy weather; it is of no use later on in a cold. There will be a lot of sneezing and a dripping, runny nose, which feels like hot water. The sufferer is restless and anxious – see Aconite in section 23 on 'Fevers' to get a full picture of the feverish kind of cold. Hepar Sulph. and Bryonia also have colds which may come on from exposure to cold, dry, windy weather. However, while Aconite is only of use for the very early stages and comes on suddenly, Hepar is particularly indicated for the later stages, and all three are very different both mentally and with the other general modalities.

Throat The throat is very inflamed and the tonsils swollen and dry. The whole throat is usually dark red in colour with burning and stinging or tingling pains.

Belladonna

Colds   This remedy is particularly useful in the early stages of a cold (Aconite, Ferrum Phos.). There is general oversensitivity to draughts, cold air, noise and light. As the eyes are sensitive to light, they are often red and watery. (Do not confuse with Arsen. Album or Euphrasia where the eyes are sore from an acrid discharge; see below.) I find that the photophobia and lachrymation, often accompanied by a slightly raised temperature, are frequently the main indicators in the early stages of a cold requiring Belladonna. The onset is always fairly sudden and symptoms usually come on from exposure to cold, wet weather (Rhus Tox.) or after getting cold suddenly when hot and sweaty. Any pains will be throbbing and pulsating, particularly if there is a headache with it. It is also useful for feverish colds (see Belladonna in section 23).

Throat   This is raw, sore, burning, very bright red and shiny (but with no ulcers or spots on it). Tonsils are swollen and it is often worse on the right side, or only on the right side. There can be hoarseness and a great sense of dryness. There is difficulty swallowing because of the dryness of the throat and Belladonna is usually very thirsty. Neck glands are often swollen too.

Ferrum Phos.

Colds   Like the Ferrum Phos. fevers and earache this remedy is of most use in the early stages but is midway in energy between the restlessness of Aconite or Belladonna and the sluggishness of Gelsemium. It is therefore a useful remedy when there are no strong symptoms pointing to other remedies, particularly Aconite or Belladonna. There is flushing alternating with pallor; indifference or dissatisfaction, and there is amelioration when alone and aggravation from interference. They are better for air and hate stuffy rooms. It is more indicated for someone who is normally fairly pale.

Bryonia

Colds   Bryonia colds come on gradually and they have extreme dryness of the lips with great thirst for long drinks. They want to lie still and be left alone as they are worse for movement and worse for company. Someone needing Bryonia for a cold will probably be very irritated by any fuss or attention. They are better for cool and worse for heating up and in hot weather. These colds can be caused by exposure to cold, dry winds (like Aconite and Hepar Sulph.) or from cooling down suddenly in hot weather. They affect the head, eyes, and nose beginning with a lot of sneezing and lachrymation, and then travel fairly quickly down to the chest (see 'Coughs', section 27).

Nux Vomica

Colds   Nux Vomica is generally worse from cold, dry weather, the slightest draught, or from fresh air. The nose runs more in the warm and gets stuffed up in cold air and at night. There is violent sneezing caused by an irritating itch in the nose. Nux Vomica never seems to be able to get warm and starts shivering on the slightest motion, draught or drinking. Mentally they are touchy and irritable (see Hepar Sulph.) and the patient will probably need Nux Vomica for his cold if he has also made you feel rather irritated with him, providing the other modalities fit.

Throat   Feels scraped, raw and sore.

Dulcamara

Colds   These colds come on when there is a change from warm weather to cold, wet weather (Rhus Tox. and Belladonna are from exposure to cold, wet weather), from exposure to snowy weather and from any sudden change in temperature. Dulcamara colds can also come on from getting wet or cold when already hot (usually in summer or autumn). The nose runs more in a warm room but there is more sneezing in the cold air. There is nearly always a stiff neck, sometimes a stiff back and limbs as well, swollen neck glands and the eyes are red and sore.

Throat   The throat can have spreading ulcers with a lot of mucus and slime generally; there may be swollen tonsils.

Rhus Tox.

Colds   These colds come on a day or so after exposure to cold, damp weather (like Belladonna, but with Belladonna the onset is fast) or from getting cold when hot and sweaty. They are worse for cold and better for warmth. (See Rhus Tox. in section 23 on 'Fevers' as well.) There may be fairly severe aching in the bones of the nose, which may have a red, sensitive tip, constant dripping as well as sneezing.

Throat   The hoarse voice is worse when first beginning to talk but then improves after talking for a little while; it then gets worse again from overuse. The throat feels raw and rough. Patients are thirsty for cold drinks although swallowing, particularly solids, is difficult, and the neck glands are often swollen.

Euphrasia

Colds   There is profuse streaming from the eyes and nose but these symptoms are opposite to Allium Cepa in that with Euphrasia the lachrymation is burning and acrid and the nasal discharge is bland. There is photophobia as with Belladonna. Many people find it difficult to describe which discharges are acrid and which are bland so it is important that you are very observant and notice where the patient looks most sore.

Allium Cepa

Colds   This remedy is for when there is profuse streaming from the eyes and nose but the lachrymation is bland and the nasal discharge is acrid. This causes soreness round the nose and above the top lip. Any sneezing and other symptoms generally are worse indoors and better for open air.

Arsen. Album

Colds   There is a thin watery nasal discharge which burns the upper lip and at the same time the nose feels blocked up; there is a lot of sneezing from irritation in the nose. This remedy is indicated for a very chilly person who likes to be wrapped up warm but needs fresh air as well. Any pains are burning and better for heat or warmth. The eyes may be dry and inflamed but there may well also be acrid lachrymation. Do not confuse this remedy with either Euphrasia or Allium Cepa; Arsen. Album has acrid discharges causing smarting and burning from *both* the nose *and* the eyes whereas with Euphrasia it is from the eyes and with Allium Cepa it is from the nose only.

Throat   This has burning pains better for warm or hot drinks.

Gelsemium

Colds   These colds come on during English summers, particularly from warm, moist weather, and develop over a few days. They also come on in winter if the weather is not particularly cold. The body feels very heavy and tired; the eyelids are droopy and half open. There is a thin, burning, watery discharge from the nose as well as a lot of sneezing. See section 23 on 'Fevers' as well so as to get a full picture of the feverish Gelsemium cold.

Throat   The tonsils are very red, may be swollen and there is difficulty swallowing because the muscles feel so weak.

Kali Bich.

Colds   The discharge is thick, stringy or ropy and also usually yellowy-green and offensive; patients hawk up thick mucus. They tend to be worse after beer and for suppressing catarrh.

Hepar Sulph.

I find this remedy always works best if you start with a 30, not lower.

Colds Only use this remedy later on in colds. It often follows an earlier remedy which has not quite finished the job. These colds come on in cold, dry weather (Aconite, Bryonia). They sweat without relief (Merc. Sol.) and sneeze a lot whenever outside in the cold (Dulcamara). There is a lot of catarrh and the discharge is usually thick and smelly. Temperamentally they are touchy, impatient and irritable (Nux Vomica). If you give this remedy too early on in a cold it appears to aggravate the condition because at best it is only partly indicated at this stage, so remember to give it only in the later stages when symptoms fit.

Throat It feels as if there is a splinter or crumb stuck in the throat (Phytolacca), and this pain is worse on swallowing. Tonsils and neck glands may be swollen.

Phytolacca

Throat This remedy has swollen tonsils and neck glands and the whole throat is dark red or bluish red; it can be covered in white/grey spots which may run together forming patches. The patient feels as if there is a lump there when swallowing (Hepar Sulph.). The pain is dry and burning particularly; there is roughness and pains may shoot to the ears on swallowing. The tongue feels burnt and/or there is pain at the root of the tongue; it can have a very red tip. They are worse swallowing anything hot and generally worse from damp, cold weather and weather changes (Rhus Tox., Dulcamara, Belladonna).

Merc. Sol.

Throat There is a raw, sore pain in the throat with the rather peculiar but very unpleasant feeling often described as an apple core scratching it. Frequently there are ulcers on the throat and tonsils and sometimes on the tongue as well. Tonsils and neck glands may be swollen. The breath will always be smelly with this remedy. There can be shooting pains from the throat into the ears as in Phytolacca and Hepar. If there is any fever there will be a lot of sweating but it will not bring any relief. They will be thirsty and there will be a lot of saliva in the mouth. Generally any symptoms are much worse at night. Always start this remedy in a 30, not lower.

Throat Gargle

A throat gargle can be made up with one teaspoon of water and a few drops of Hypercal Ø in it. (Hypercal is a mixture of equal parts of Hypericum Ø and Calendula Ø.) It does not taste very nice and stings a bit, but it works as a kind of antiseptic and can be a great help. Remember that most ordinary mouthwashes contain substances which antidote homoeopathic remedies (see pages 23–25) and should not be used.

A BRIEF SUMMARY OF THE MAIN INDICATIONS FOR REMEDIES FOR COLDS AND SORE THROATS

The following is a summary of the **strongly indicated symptoms only** for the remedies described above. If you check through these as well as read up the remedy pictures in this section and in the Materia Medica in chapter six, it should make it easier for you to choose. For really nasty sore throats also check through the remedy summary in the section 42 on 'Diphtheria' as it gives a wider selection of throat remedy details (this does not mean you could have diphtheria!).

Alone ameliorates:	Ferrum Phos., Bryonia
Anxious:	Aconite
Appearance, nose tip red:	Rhus Tox.
Appearance, tongue tip red:	Rhus Tox., Phyt.
Back stiff:	Dulc., Rhus Tox.

Body temperature, cannot get warm:	Nux Vom., Bell.
Breath smelly:	Merc. Sol.
Caused by change from warm to cold wet weather:	Dulc., Phyt., Rhus Tox.
Caused by cold dry windy:	Aconite, Bryonia
Caused by cold raw dry:	Aconite, Bryonia, Hepar Sulph., Nux Vom.
Caused by cold wet:	Bell., Rhus Tox.
Caused by cooling suddenly in hot weather:	Bryonia
Caused by getting cold and wet/damp:	Bell., Rhus Tox., Phyt.
Caused by getting cold and/or wet when hot:	Dulc., Rhus Tox., Bell.
Caused by getting cold when hot/sweaty:	Bell., Rhus Tox., Dulc.
Caused by warm weather, summer:	Gels.
Caused by warm wet weather:	Gels.
Caused by warm winter weather:	Gels.
Chilly on slightest motion:	Nux Vom.
Company aggravates:	Bryonia, Ferrum Phos.
Dissatisfaction:	Ferrum Phos.
Dryness, lips:	Bryonia
Dryness, throat:	Aconite, Bell., Bryonia, Phyt.
Early stages:	Aconite, Bell., Ferrum Phos.
Energy completely lacking:	Gels.
Eyes, discharge acrid:	Euph., Arsen. Album
Eyes, droopy lids, can hardly keep open:	Gels.
Eyes, dry:	Arsen. Album
Eyes, profuse discharge:	Euph., Allium Cepa, Arsen. Album

Eyes, red:	Bell., Dulc., Arsen. Album
Eyes, watery:	Bell., Bryonia, Euph., Allium Cepa
Face flushing alternating with pallor:	Ferrum Phos., Aconite
Feverish particularly:	Aconite, Bell., Ferrum Phos.
Glands neck swollen:	Dulc., Bell., Bryonia, Rhus Tox., Phyt., Hepar Sulph., Merc. Sol., Kali Bich.
Impatient and touchy:	Hepar Sulph., Nux Vom.
Indifference:	Ferrum Phos.
Interference aggravates:	Ferrum Phos., Bryonia, Nux Vom.
Irritable:	Nux Vom., Hepar Sulph.
Irritated by fuss and attention:	Ferrum Phos., Bryonia
Later stages in cold:	Hepar Sulph., Kali Bich.
Limbs stiff:	Dulc., Rhus Tox.
Lips, sore top lip and below nose:	Allium Cepa, Arsen. Album
Motion aggravates:	Bryonia, Nux Vom.
Neck stiff:	Dulc., Rhus Tox.
Night, symptoms worse:	Merc. Sol.
Noise aggravates:	Bell.
Nose, bones ache:	Rhus Tox.
Nose, constant dripping:	Rhus Tox.
Nose, discharge acrid and burning:	Allium Cepa, Arsen. Album, Gels.

Nose, discharge bland:	Euph., Pulsatilla
Nose, discharge like hot water:	Aconite
Nose, discharge smelly:	Hepar Sulph., Merc. Sol., Kali Bich.
Nose, discharge stringy and ropy:	Kali Bich.
Nose, discharge thick:	Kali Bich., Pulsatilla, Hepar Sulph.
Nose, discharge yellow-green-white:	Kali Bich., Pulsatilla, Hepar Sulph.
Nose, discharge profuse watery:	Euph., Allium Cepa, Arsen. Album, Gels.
Nose, stuffed up at night:	Nux Vom.
Nose, stuffed up in cold air:	Nux Vom.
Nose, stuffed up:	Arsen. Album, Nux Vom., Pulsatilla (worse warm room)
Nose, watery discharge in warm room:	Nux Vom., Dulc.
Onset slow:	Bryonia, Rhus Tox.
Onset sudden:	Aconite, Bell., Ferrum Phos.
Pains, aching of bones of nose:	Rhus Tox.
Pains, at root of tongue:	Phyt.
Pains, burning better for warmth:	Arsen. Album
Pains, feels heavy and tired and no energy:	Gels.
Pains, throbbing and pulsating:	Bell.
Pale type usually:	Ferrum Phos.
Photophobia:	Bell., Euph.
Restless:	Aconite, Bell., Rhus Tox., Arsen. Album
Saliva increased:	Merc. Sol.

Side left:	Rhus Tox.
Side right:	Bell.
Sluggish:	Gels.
Sneezing a lot:	Aconite, Bryonia, Nux Vom., Rhus Tox., Arsen. Album, Gels.
Sneezing from irritating itch in nose:	Nux Vom., Arsen. Album, Pulsatilla
Sneezing in cold air:	Dulc., Hepar Sulph.
Sneezing worse indoors:	Allium Cepa
Speed, cold travels quickly to chest:	Bryonia
Stiffness in back and limbs:	Dulc., Rhus Tox.
Stuffy rooms aggravate:	Ferrum Phos., Pulsatilla
Swallowing, difficult:	Bell., Gels., Hepar Sulph., Rhus Tox. (solids particularly)
Swallowing, warm drinks ameliorate:	Arsen. Album
Swallowing, warm/hot things aggravate:	Phyt.
Sweats without relief:	Hepar Sulph., Merc. Sol.
Thirst for cold drinks:	Rhus Tox.
Thirst for milk:	Rhus Tox.
Thirsty:	Bell., Merc. Sol., Phyt.
Throat colour bluish-red:	Phyt.
Throat colour bright red:	Bell.
Throat colour dark red:	Aconite, Phyt.
Throat covered in mucus and slime:	Dulc.
Throat covered in white/grey patches:	Phyt.
Throat covered in white/grey spots:	Phyt.
Throat dry particularly:	Aconite, Bell., Phyt., Bryonia

Throat hawks up thick mucus:	Kali Bich., Merc. Sol., Hepar Sulph.
Throat pain as if apple core scratching it:	Merc. Sol.
Throat pain as if scraped:	Nux Vom.
Throat pain better for warm drinks:	Arsen. Album, Hepar Sulph.
Throat pain burning:	Aconite, Bell., Arsen. Album, Phyt.
Throat pain feels rough:	Rhus Tox., Phyt.
Throat pain like a lump when swallowing:	Phyt., Hepar Sulph.
Throat pain like a splinter or crumb:	Hepar Sulph., Phyt., Merc. Sol.
Throat pain raw and sore:	Bell., Nux Vom., Rhus Tox., Merc. Sol.
Throat pain stinging:	Aconite
Throat pain tingling:	Aconite
Throat pains shoot to ears:	Phyt., Hepar Sulph., Merc. Sol.
Throat shining:	Bell.
Throat ulcers with a cold:	Merc. Sol., Hepar Sulph., Kali Bich., Arsen. Album, Dulc.
Tongue, feels burnt:	Phyt.
Tongue, pain at root:	Phyt.
Tongue, tip sensitive:	Rhus Tox.
Tongue, triangular tip red:	Rhus Tox., Phyt.
Tonsils red:	Bell., Gels.
Tonsils swollen generally:	Dulc., Aconite, Bell., Nux Vom., Merc. Sol., Gels., Kali Bich., Hepar Sulph., Phyt.

Touchy:	Nux Vom., Hepar Sulph.
Voice hoarse worse from overuse:	Rhus Tox.
Voice hoarse worse initial speaking:	Rhus Tox.
Weakness extreme:	Gels., Arsen. Album
Weather, worse for changes to cool, worse autumn:	Dulc.
Weather, fresh air ameliorates:	Ferrum Phos., Pulsatilla, Allium Cepa
Weather, warm aggravates:	Gels.
Weather, warm and wet aggravates:	Gels.
Weather, warm winter weather aggravates:	Gels.
Weather/room temperature, better for cool air:	Aconite, Bryonia, Arsen. Album (head only), Allium Cepa
Weather/room temperature, worse cold air:	Bell., Nux Vom., Rhus Tox., Hepar Sulph., Arsen. Album
Weather/room temperature, worse draughts:	Bell., Nux Vom., Rhus Tox., Hepar Sulph.
Weather/room temperature, worse for warmth:	Aconite, Bryonia, Allium Cepa
Weather/room temperature, better for warmth:	Rhus Tox., Arsen. Album, Bell., Hepar Sulph.

25. Earache

There are many remedies for earache and it often accompanies fevers and other illnesses. If the patient does not respond fairly quickly to the remedy you have given, it means the illness is probably more complicated than it at first seems and prescribing for it is beyond the scope of this book. If this is the case you must consult a professional homoeopath at once. Both acute and chronic homoeopathic treatment for ear problems should usually prevent the need for children to have grommets inserted, as well as help in preventing other possible hearing complications.

There are three main remedies to consider for acute otitis media which should usually prevent more serious symptoms developing. Since earache so often accompanies fevers and colds it may help you to get a complete picture of these three remedies if you also read their descriptions in sections 23 and 24, on 'Fevers', 'Colds and sore throats', as well as in the Materia Medica.

Aconite

The Aconite earache comes on suddenly after exposure to cold, dry, windy weather. It will usually be worse in the evening at about 9 pm. Again, like Ferrum Phos., it is useful in the first stages of earache. The ear is red, hot, dry and painful, and the sufferer will be extremely restless and fearful. When well the Aconite type is more likely to have ruddy cheeks and seem quite strong and healthy, quite different from the pale, easily tired Ferrum Phos. type.

Belladonna

This remedy again has sudden onset but unlike Aconite it is after exposure to cold, wet, windy weather and is worse at around 3 am and/or 3 pm. Patients are irritable, cross and grumpy rather than fearful like Aconite. The ear and surrounding area will probably be red, hot, dry and burning, but under the hair and the clothes they will be sweaty. It usually affects the right ear, or the right ear is the worst ear, but if the other symptoms fit, Belladonna will cure even if it is only the left ear that is affected. They will be hypersensitive to noise, light, and draughts.

Ferrum Phos.

This remedy is most frequently indicated in the early stages of earache. Its symptoms are not particularly distinctive but there is an alternation between being flushed or pale generally on the face and sometimes on the ear itself; this symptom is easy to miss unless you are very observant. It is used for both mild and more violent earache. The onset is sudden with a dull but fairly persistent ache, accompanied by local congestion and inflammation. As mentioned, Ferrum Phos. is most useful in the early stages and if taken then, when symptoms indicate it, it will probably be the only remedy needed, preventing more serious problems. It is particularly suited for those who are rather pale when well and may tend to get tired easily.

The following remedies should be considered for earaches which have less acute inflammation and less visible redness to the area, but are more likely to have discharges; pains may easily be as severe.

Merc. Sol.

Although this earache may come on suddenly there is not much inflammation compared to Belladonna, Aconite or Ferrum Phos. There may be a thick, yellow, bloody discharge but the main feature is that the pains are shooting and may come from the throat or from the teeth into the ear and are sharp. Discharges are always smelly and breath will be offensive. If there is any fever there will be sweating but without any relief from it. There may be profuse saliva but there will be great thirst as well. Pain and symptoms will probably be worse at night. Always start this remedy in a 30, not lower, and improvement should start within ten minutes or so.

Hepar Sulph.

Again like Merc. Sol. there is not much inflammation when compared to Aconite, Belladonna or Ferrum Phos. Like Merc. Sol. there can be suppuration and discharges may be smelly; pains are darting, sticking or splinter-like in the ear. They are worse for cold, draughts and uncovering. Mentally they are impatient, touchy and oversensitive. The symptoms are most likely to come on after exposure to cold dry air.

Pulsatilla

This earache is worse in the evening and night and usually is caused by catarrh blocking the eustachian tubes. The ear may be red and swollen, and may feel as if something is pushing outwards with a kind of pressing pain. They may have a dry mouth but are seldom if ever thirsty. They can overheat quite easily and hate stuffy rooms. Mentally they may be tearful and they do not want to be left alone.

26. Croup

Usually only young children suffer from croup and it is an illness they tend to grow out of. However while it is happening it can be very unpleasant and quite alarming. Homoeopathy is extremely helpful and usually one of the three acute remedies below will bring dramatic relief for your child. All these croup remedies are worse for dryness and better for wet and damp.

Aconite

Use Aconite if the symptoms start in the early evening, until about midnight; occasionally they can recur at about 9 am. The croup symptoms will often come on after exposure to cold, dry, windy weather, or after a fright. Your child will be very frightened, anxious and restless, throwing off the bedclothes, feeling better for uncovering and worse in a warm room. There will be dry wheezing and a tight feeling in the chest. The cough is dry, short, barking or whistling. The child grasps his throat while trying to get his breath. There may also be fever with sudden onset, the skin being red, hot, dry and burning and there is great thirst as well. The red face can go quite pale when they sit or stand up.

I find it is best to start with Aconite 30 particularly as there is usually a lot of fear, anxiety and restlessness. You may need to give the remedy every few minutes for the first few doses but, as always, follow the 'Rules about dosage, potencies and repetition of doses' in section 10. Quite often your child will feel better after only one or two doses.

Spongia

If your child is not improving, or relapses badly within about one hour or so after starting the Aconite, you should go on to Spongia. Spongia is indicated when the symptoms are worse from just before midnight until early in the morning, about 4 am. The Spongia croup has a dry, barking cough sounding like a 'saw driven through wood'. Spongia is worse lying and better sitting bent forward, and the croupy symptoms may start while they are asleep, waking them up with a sense of suffocation. They are worse for cold drinks and better for anything warm; also worse for sweets. I usually start with Spongia 6 but quite frequently have to go up to Spongia 30.

Hepar Sulph.

This remedy is particularly useful when the croup comes on or becomes worse again in the early hours of the morning, as well as from exposure to dry, cold wind. By the early hours of the morning the cough, though still sounding croupy, is somewhat looser. There can be rattling in the chest with wheezing but they are unable to cough up any mucus. They are worse for cold air and uncovering and better for warmth, heat and damp weather. Mentally they are touchy, irritable and impatient. Start with Hepar Sulph. 30.

27. Coughs

I am dividing coughs into dry coughs and loose-sounding coughs with a lot of mucus in the chest. The following remedies are only a few of a vast number which help in these complaints and should only be used in the acute disease. It must be remembered that if someone is prone to getting bronchitis or other chest problems then a qualified professional homoeopath should be consulted. This is so that they can have deeper constitutional treatment, thus reducing the tendency to get sick in the first place. Please remember that most ordinary cough mixtures and cough sweets usually contain substances which antidote homoeopathic remedies; such as menthol, eucalyptus etc. (see pages 23–25). You must avoid taking these or there will be no point taking the homoeopathic remedy; you can always make up a soothing mixture of warm honey and lemon if necessary, but you should find that the homoeopathic remedy brings relief fairly quickly.

DRY COUGHS

Aconite

The Aconite dry cough will often come on after exposure to cold, dry, windy weather or after a fright. The cough is dry, short, barking or whistling. Sufferers grasp their throat while trying to get their breath. They are worse in a warm room, better if uncovered, better for expiration and possibly worse about 9 pm. Mentally they are very restless, very frightened and anxious. There is dryness and a tight, possibly hot feeling in the chest, and there is little or no expectoration. The cough can occur while they sleep and sometimes wakes them.

Spongia

Spongia has a dry barking cough sounding like a 'saw driven through wood'. They are worse lying, better sitting bent forward, and the cough may come on during sleep and wake them up with a sense of suffocation, which may well frighten them. There is a definite time aggravation from before midnight until the early hours of the morning, so for someone prone to getting Spongia coughs this is the most likely time that they will be disturbed in the night; it is a good idea to give someone with this kind of cough an extra pillow. They are worse for cold drinks, better for anything warm and worse for sweets. There may be hoarseness. Although initially the chest is dry and there is no mucus, later on there can be tough mucus which is hard to expectorate.

Belladonna

With the Belladonna cough there is great dryness in the larynx, which gets worse and worse until a burning, tickling, scraping sensation causes the cough. The cough itself is very hard and frequent, continuing until a tiny bit of mucus is raised, which makes them feel a little better until the dryness of the throat starts it all off again. Remember the typical Belladonna picture is of redness, burning heat, dilated pupils, possible lachrymation, worse for light, for noise, at 3 pm or 3 am and for draughts, and better sitting half propped. They may cough while asleep.

Bryonia

This is a hard dry cough with soreness and stitching pains in the chest and the cough shakes the whole body. It often follows a head cold which has travelled fairly quickly down to the chest. Bryonia is worse from cold dry weather, worse in an east wind, worse for motion and better for pressure; so you see the sufferer sitting very still with his arms hugging or pressing against his chest. Bryonia is always thirsty, worse for hot weather or in a warm room, better for cool air and damp days and better left alone. Their cough is also worse from sighing or taking a deep breath, may be worse at about 9 pm and sometimes is loose in the morning.

Ferrum Phos.

This cough is dry, short or hacking and may accompany inflammation and congestion of the lungs. Ferrum Phos. desires air and the cough is much worse in a stuffy or hot room. There can be pain on both sides of the chest. Sometimes they may cough up some blood. They can feel weak and exhausted and can alternate between being flushed or pale.

Causticum

This cough is dry and there is a feeling of rawness and dryness all the way down from the throat to the chest. The chest itself feels full of mucus and they feel that if only they could cough a little deeper they could get some mucus up. They are generally unable to expectorate but, if they do, it always slips back down again. The cough is worse on expiration. There can be escape of urine, or pain in the hip, during the cough, and they find that sips of cold water give them some relief. Generally they are better for wet weather and warmth, and worse in dry weather, windy weather and draughts. There may be hoarseness, which is worse in the morning. The cough may waken them from sleep and it is very much worse lying down. For people with a Causticum cough it is always a good idea to give them an extra pillow or two at night so they are not lying so flat.

Phosphorus

This cough is worse in open air and from going from warm to cold or vice versa. It is a dry, tickling cough with irritation behind the sternum (breastbone) or in the larynx, it can also be so violent that it racks them and they may hold onto their chest (as does Bryonia). It is often worse from twilight until about midnight, worse lying on the left side and better lying on the right, worse when talking and eating and worse when left alone. They crave cold things such as ice cream and cold water although they themselves are chilly. There is a sense of a great weight lying on the chest, of constriction. The larynx may be very painful and worse from talking; the voice may be hoarse and gets worse in the evening; expectoration may be bloody. They may cough during sleep or it may wake them from sleep.

Rhus Tox.

This dry cough is from a tickle usually behind the upper sternum (breastbone) or else from the slightest uncovering such as putting a hand out from under the bedclothes. It is worse from cold, wet weather, or from getting cold or cooling down too quickly when still hot and sweaty from exertion. They are very restless and cough in their sleep, or it may prevent sleep. There may be hoarseness which is worse for initial talking, but improves after a while if they continue talking.

Drosera

This cough is from violent tickling in the larynx and they go on and on coughing in paroxysms till they retch or vomit. It feels as if the cough is coming from deep down in the chest. They are worse after midnight until the early hours of the morning, worse lying down and are somewhat better if given an extra pillow. They may hold the chest when coughing (Bryonia and Phosphorus) which is worse when talking, laughing, eating and drinking; there may be some hoarseness. The cough may waken them from sleep. The nose may bleed from the violence of the cough and they are better for fresh air.

Rumex

This cough is worse from the slightest exposure to cold air and very much worse for inspiration. People who need Rumex will walk around when outside with a scarf covering their mouth so as to stop themselves breathing in the cold air. Rumex is worse just moving from a warm to a colder room. There is a constant tickle in the throat feeling like dust which leads to a dry, teasing cough; despite this there is a lot of expectoration and mucus with a desire to hawk, which does not relieve. There may be leaking of urine with each cough. It is very much worse lying down so you should give them an extra pillow.

LOOSE AND DRY COUGHS

Pulsatilla

Although this cough is mostly loose, it is also changeable in that it may be dryer in the evening and looser in the morning. The other main feature is that the cough is worse on warming up, worse when entering a warm room or getting overheated. The Pulsatilla type is always opening the windows in order to get some fresh air and cool down, although, just to be confusing, when acutely ill they can be chilly. Pulsatilla is thirstless like Ipecac. and Antim. Tart. Any expectoration is thick, bland and yellow/green.

OTHER CHANGEABLE COUGHS

Bryonia, see Dry Coughs, can sound loose in mornings, but is usually dry. Causticum and Rumex, see Dry Coughs, can both have a lot of mucus in the chest but the cough itself sounds dry. Ipecac., see Loose Sounding Coughs, can sound dry occasionally. Hepar Sulph., see Loose Sounding Coughs, can sound dryer at night.

LOOSE SOUNDING COUGHS WITH A LOT OF MUCUS IN THE CHEST

Hepar Sulph.

This cough often follows the end of a bad head cold. It is loose, deep and rough and there is rattling in the chest although it is fairly difficult to cough up any mucus; if they do, the mucus is thick and yellow. They are worse for cold air and better for warmth and damp weather. The cough is worse whenever any part of the body is uncovered as with Rhus Tox. Symptoms may come on from cold, dry, windy weather. There may be hoarseness and the cough can be dryer during the night.

Antim. Tart.

This is a particularly loose cough with a great deal of rattling in the chest. They have difficulty coughing anything up and it sounds as if they are drowning in mucus. It is especially useful for coughs of very young children and the elderly, so you may find it useful quite often while your children are very small as well as for your parents or grandparents. They are better sitting, worse for heat and worse when the bedclothes make them too warm. They are usually completely thirstless. These coughs are worse in damp weather, in autumn and living in damp places. If they do feel nauseous they are better for vomiting. Their face can have a blue tinge particularly round the nose and mouth.

Ipecac.

This cough is very like Antim. Tart. in that there is a lot of mucus in the chest with difficult expectoration (although the cough may sound either dry and croupy, or loose and rattly). They can just manage to cough up some mucus when the cough is violent and goes on and on (Drosera). They are thirstless and worse for damp weather like Antim. Tart., better for fresh air and better for warmth. However, with Ipecac. they often feel nauseous, they are no better for vomiting and if you look at the tongue it will be clean not coated. They may cough up blood.

Kali Bich.

This cough remedy is noted for the ropy, stringy mucus, which they manage to cough up. They are better for expectoration and there may be hoarseness, which is worse in the evening. They may point to a particular place in their throat where a tickle or rawness starts off the cough. They may constantly be clearing the throat.

A BRIEF SUMMARY OF THE MAIN INDICATIONS FOR COUGH REMEDIES

The following is a summary of the **strongly indicated symptoms only** for the remedies described above. If you check through these as well as read up the remedy pictures in this section and in the Materia Medica in chapter six, it should make it easier for you to choose.

Air ameliorates:	Ferrum Phos., Pulsatilla, Ipecac., Dros.
Alone aggravates:	Phos., Pulsatilla,
Anxious:	Aconite
Appearance alternates between flushed and pale:	Ferrum Phos., Aconite
Appearance has a blue tinge round nose and/or mouth:	Antim. Tart.
Appearance has a clean tongue despite nausea:	Ipecac.
Appetite craves cold things:	Phos.
Breathing deeply aggravates:	Bryonia
Caused by a bad head cold:	Hepar Sulph., Bryonia
Caused by a fright:	Aconite
Caused by a tickle in throat:	Bell., Phos., Rhus Tox., Dros., Rumex, Kali Bich.
Caused by cold dry windy:	Aconite, Bryonia, Caust., Rumex, Hepar Sulph.
Caused by cold wet:	Bell., Rhus Tox.
Caused by cooling suddenly in hot weather:	Bryonia
Caused by extreme dryness in throat:	Bell.

Caused by getting cold and wet or damp: Bell., Rhus Tox.

Caused by getting cold and/or wet if
hot and/or sweaty: Rhus Tox., Bell.

Caused by head cold travelling fast to
lungs: Bryonia

Caused by living in damp places: Antim. Tart.

Caused by scraping feeling in throat: Bell.

Caused by throat burning: Bell.

Caused by tickle in throat in one
particular place: Kali Bich.

Changeable coughs, sounding loose
and/or dry: Pulsatilla, Bryonia,
Hepar Sulph.

Children and babies with loose sounding
coughs: Antim. Tart.

Cold, craves cold things although chilly: Phos.

Coughs barking: Aconite, Spongia

Coughs deep: Hepar Sulph.

Coughs from a feeling of dust in throat: Rumex

Coughs from draughts: Bell., Caust., Rhus Tox.,
Hepar Sulph.

Coughs from tickle behind sternum: Phos., Rhus Tox.

Coughs from tickle in throat: Bell., Phos., Rhus Tox.,
Dros., Rumex,
Kali Bich.

Coughs, paroxysms on and on without
pause: Dros., Ipecac.

Coughs rough: Hepar Sulph.

Coughs till vomits: Dros., Ipecac.

Coughs particularly violent: Phos., Bryonia, Dros.,
Ipecac.

Drinking aggravates:	Bryonia, Dros.
Drinks a lot at a time, always thirsty:	Bryonia, Phos.
Drinks, cold drinks aggravate:	Spongia
Drinks, cold things, very thirsty:	Phos.
Drinks, sips of water ameliorate:	Caust.
Drinks, warm drinks ameliorate:	Spongia
Dry and loose sounding coughs:	Bryonia, Pulsatilla, Hepar Sulph.
Dry sounding coughs with much mucus in chest:	Caust., Rumex, (sometimes Ipecac. can sound dry although usually sounds loose)
Dry sounding coughs:	Aconite, Spongia, Bell., Bryonia, Ferrum Phos., Caust., Phos., Rhus Tox., Dros., Rumex, Pulsatilla (changeable), Ipecac. (usually sounds loose)
Eating aggravates:	Phos., Bryonia, Dros.
Elderly people with loose sounding coughs:	Antim. Tart.
Expectoration, ropy and stringy:	Kali Bich.
Expectoration, bloody:	Ferrum Phos., Phos., Ipecac.
Expectoration, cannot cough deep enough to raise:	Caust.
Expectoration, difficult at first, easier later on:	Hepar Sulph., Spongia
Expectoration, difficult, eventually a tiny bit:	Bell.

Expectoration, difficult:	Caust., Antim. Tart., Ipecac., Phos., Rumex
Expectoration, profuse despite dry sounding cough:	Rumex
Expectoration, slips back down if raised:	Caust.
Expectoration, thick:	Pulsatilla, Hepar Sulph., Kali Bich.
Expectoration, yellow green:	Pulsatilla, Hepar Sulph., Kali Bich.
Frightened:	Aconite, Spongia
Grasp throat on coughing and breathing:	Aconite
Hawks up mucus frequently:	Rumex, Kali Bich.
Hoarseness worse in the evening:	Phos.
Hoarseness worse in the morning:	Caust., Rhus Tox.
Hoarseness worse initial talking, better continued:	Rhus Tox.
Hoarseness:	Spongia, Rhus Tox., Phos., Caust., Dros., Hepar Sulph., Kali Bich.
Later stages, some mucus, difficult to expectorate:	Spongia, Hepar Sulph.
Laughing aggravates:	Bryonia, Dros.
Loose and dry sounding coughs, alternating:	Pulsatilla, Bryonia, Hepar Sulph.
Loose sounding coughs:	Hepar Sulph., Antim. Tart., Ipecac., Kali Bich., Pulsatilla
Motion aggravates:	Bryonia
Mucus profuse in lungs:	Antim. Tart., Ipecac., Caust., Rumex, Pulsatilla, Hepar Sulph.

COMMON ACUTE AILMENTS

Nausea, better for vomiting:	Antim. Tart.
Nausea, no better for vomiting:	Ipecac.
Nosebleed from violence of cough:	Dros., (sometimes Pulsatilla), Ipecac.
Overheating aggravates:	Pulsatilla
Pains, chest better for firm pressure and/or holding:	Bryonia
Pains, as if great weight on chest:	Phos.
Pains, both sides of chest:	Ferrum Phos.
Pains, constriction of chest:	Phos., Aconite
Pains, in chest stitching:	Bryonia
Pains, in hip with cough:	Caust.
Pains, raw and dry all the way down to chest:	Caust.
Position, better lying on right side:	Phos.
Position, holds chest because cough so violent:	Phos., Bryonia, Dros.
Position, lying aggravates:	Spongia, Caust., Dros., Rumex, Antim. Tart., Bryonia, Pulsatilla, Rhus Tox., Phos.
Position, must sit up:	Antim. Tart., Phos., Pulsatilla, Bryonia, Dros., Kali Bich.
Position, sits hugging or pressing arms against chest:	Bryonia, Dros., Phos.
Position, sitting bent forward ameliorates:	Spongia
Position, worse lying on left side:	Phos.
Rattling of mucus in chest:	Hepar Sulph., Ipecac., Antim. Tart., Pulsatilla
Restless:	Aconite, Rhus Tox.

Shaking of body during cough:	Bryonia
Sighing aggravates:	Bryonia
Sweets aggravate:	Spongia
Talking aggravates:	Bryonia, Phos., Dros.
Thirstless:	Pulsatilla, Ipecac., Antim. Tart.
Time, coming on during sleep:	Spongia, Bell., Caust., Phos., Rhus Tox., Dros.
Time, cough wakes them from sleep:	Phos., Spongia, Dros., Caust.
Time, looser in day and dryer at night:	Pulsatilla, Hepar Sulph.
Time, waking from sleep with suffocating feel:	Spongia
Time, worse 9 pm:	Aconite, Bryonia
Time, worse around 3 pm and 3 am:	Bell.
Time, worse before midnight until early hours of morning:	Spongia
Time, worse from about midnight till early hours:	Dros.
Time, worse in evening:	Kali Bich., Phos., Pulsatilla
Time, worse twilight until about midnight:	Phos.
Uncovering aggravates:	Rhus Tox., Hepar Sulph.
Urination involuntary with cough:	Caust., Rumex
Weak and exhausted:	Ferrum Phos.
Weather, fresh air ameliorates:	Ferrum Phos., Pulsatilla, Ipecac.
Weather, warm wet ameliorates:	Caust., Hepar Sulph., Bryonia
Weather, wet aggravates:	Antim. Tart., Rhus Tox., Bell., Ipecac.

Weather, worse autumn:	Antim. Tart.
Weather, worse cold wet:	Bell., Rhus Tox.
Weather/room temperature, worse going from cold to hot:	Phos., Bryonia
Weather/room temperature, worse going from hot to cold:	Phos., Rumex
Weather/room temperature, better for cool air:	Aconite, Bryonia, Ferrum Phos., Pulsatilla
Weather/room temperature, worse change of:	Phos.
Weather/room temperature, worse cold air:	Bell., Rhus Tox., Phos., Hepar Sulph., Rumex
Weather/room temperature, worse draughts:	Bell., Rhus Tox., Caust., Hepar Sulph., Rumex
Weather/room temperature, worse warmth:	Aconite, Bryonia, Ferrum Phos., Pulsatilla, Antim. Tart.
Weather/room temperature, better warmth:	Rhus Tox., Bell., Hepar Sulph., Ipecac.

28. Digestive problems: food poisoning, overeating, acute diarrhoea and colic

All of the remedies in this section should be considered when someone has acute diarrhoea. There are many remedies for these conditions, but the remedies described in this section are the ones most commonly indicated. The remedies most frequently needed for digestive problems associated with teething are Chamomilla, Podophyllum and Ipecac. For chronic digestive problems, or if the acute remedy does not help, you must consult your homoeopath.

FOOD POISONING

Arsen. Album

This remedy is for food poisoning from drinking dirty water, eating badly washed vegetables (or vegetables washed in dirty water), watery fruits and cold foods. It can be from eating bad meat as well (see Pyrogen below) if the symptoms fit, but this is less common. With Arsen. Album there is vomiting and diarrhoea at the same time. Any pains are burning but they are better for warmth and hot applications. There is a time aggravation at midnight or soon after. There is burning unquenchable thirst but they only have sips each time. They may crave cold water but vomit this straight away because they are worse for anything cold to eat or drink. They are fearful and restless, sometimes thinking they are going to die and that it is pointless to take any medicine; they do not want to be left on their own. They are also critical and exacting. Despite being sweaty, weak, very cold, and wanting warmth, they want fresh air as well, insisting on having the window open and their head near the window if possible. They are incredibly weak and prostrated, and all their suffering seems to you as you observe them to be out of proportion to the actual symptoms.

Pyrogen

This remedy is for food poisoning from eating bad fish or meat. The main symptom is that all discharges (stools, sweat) have a disgusting smell and the breath and mouth are offensive too. There is intense aching in the bones, restlessness and wriggling, the sufferer being momentarily better for motion. They are better for hot drinks or a hot bath. The pulse is abnormally rapid, out of proportion to any fever. They are conscious of the heart beating.

OVEREATING

Pulsatilla

This remedy is for overeating rich foods such as cream, fat, pastries, cakes and so on. Pulsatilla types frequently want to eat the very foods which make them ill. They are usually thirstless, even with a dry mouth; they need fresh air, are better for cold applications, are worse for warmth and worse in the evening. Any pains are changeable; that is they move around changing from place to place, and the type of pain varies too. If there is diarrhoea the stools vary each time and these symptoms are usually worse at night. Pulsatilla always feels better for walking gently and slowly around in cool, open air. Temperamentally they are mild, gentle and weepy, disliking being alone and enjoying any attention they may get.

Nux Vomica

This remedy is useful for digestive pains following overeating of rich, or spicy, highly seasoned foods, such as curries. Mentally they feel very irritable and can be impatient, bad tempered and angry. They are oversensitive, touchy, easily offended and worse in the early morning, as well as being worse for noise, odours, and touch. People who need Nux Vomica behave very like someone with a hangover, and Nux Vomica is the main remedy for hangovers. Nux Vomica types are usually very organized; the milder tempered ones are less irritable but more worried about everything around them being orderly. Nausea and stomach pains are better for vomiting and hot drinks; there is diarrhoea with a lot of fruitless urging and a 'never-get-done' feeling. There is often a sensation of pressure, or of a weight like a stone in the stomach. Symptoms tend to occur an hour or two after eating.

Ipecac.

This is a remedy for diarrhoea which can occur from overeating rich food, sweets or fruit, or while your child is teething. The symptoms can also come on from reserved displeasure or indignation such as when people think they have been scolded or treated unfairly. Stools can be fermenting, grass green, or watery, slimy, bloody or with a lot of mucus. Nausea is always persistent with this remedy and there is no relief from vomiting; there may be bright red blood when vomiting. The tongue is always clean which is very unusual accompanying these kinds of digestive symptoms. There is no thirst.

ACUTE DIARRHOEA

You must also consider Arsen. Album, Pyrogen, Pulsatilla, Nux Vomica, and Ipecac, mentioned above, any of which could be needed for someone with acute diarrhoea. The danger of acute diarrhoea is dehydration (particularly for children) and you can always make sure this is avoided by giving them Dioralyte from your local pharmacy; if you prefer, you could make up a solution yourself with water, honey or sugar and a small amount of sea salt. On the whole however, the homoeopathic remedies usually work fast enough for such precautions to be unnecessary. China 6 or Phos. Ac. 6 are also useful remedies to take if there has been loss of fluids.

Aconite

This is a remedy for diarrhoea which comes on during hot weather (see Podophyllum below), particularly when the days are hot and the nights cool; also from exposure to cold, dry, windy weather. Stools are slimy, green, bloody, white or watery. Patients are extremely restless, thirsty and fearful. Colic pains force them to bend double but there is no relief from this at all.

Bryonia

This is a remedy for diarrhoea which occurs during hot weather, particularly after eating or drinking cold things when very hot. It is worse for cooling down suddenly when already hot. The colicky pains are better for pressure so sufferers double up. Diarrhoea and any pains are worse on the slightest movement and worse in the morning. There is a sensation of heaviness and weight in the stomach (Nux Vomica). The mouth and lips are very dry and patients are extremely thirsty, drinking large quantities at a time.

Chamomilla

Mentally the Chamomilla type is extremely angry, restless and impatient and this remedy should be considered whenever there is extreme anger with any pain, whatever the cause of the pain may be. Stools are often green and look like chopped spinach, or else yellowy in colour; they smell like rotten eggs. The abdomen is often distended and the pains are cutting, causing sufferers to toss about in agony. The abdominal pains are better for warmth although any tooth and gum pains are better for cold drinks. There is thirst as well as a lot of dribbling and saliva. This remedy should also be considered for diarrhoea as well as colic which occur particularly when a baby is teething, (see Chamomilla in section 29).

Dulcamara

This remedy is for diarrhoea and colic following exposure to cold wet weather, or from cooling down suddenly when hot, and any sudden weather changes. It is particularly indicated in autumn with warmish days, which suddenly get cold in the late afternoon or early evening. Stools are slimy, mucousy and watery; they can be greenish or yellow in colour. There is cramping or griping pain around the navel. Symptoms tend to be worse at night.

Podophyllum

This is an excellent remedy for diarrhoea which comes on during hot summer weather. There is a lot of noisy rumbling and gurgling in the abdomen before the stool. The diarrhoea is worse early in the morning but by evening is usually considerably better. The stools are green, chalky, foaming, watery, white, or with a yellow sediment; they are very smelly, profuse and gushing. It is usually painless but afterwards they may feel sore and weak. The liver area is swollen and sore and is better for rubbing. They are worse for acid fruits and for milk and worse during teething. The face may be yellowish or else flushed. They are probably very restless and roll the head from side to side and/or grind the teeth. Like Chamomilla and Ipecac. this is a remedy which should be considered when babies get diarrhoea during teething (see Podophyllum in section 29).

Phos. Ac.

This remedy is indicated when there is extreme weakness and debility but no actual pain from the diarrhoea. Alternatively it can be indicated when the diarrhoea has gone on for some time but *without* actually weakening them. The diarrhoea is always painless, very watery and seldom smelly; this remedy is also well indicated if children have been growing fast. Like China it is useful when there has been loss of fluids; for this give it in a 6 three times a day for a few days.

COLIC

For treating colic you should also consider Arsen. Album, Pulsatilla, Nux Vomica, Aconite, Podophyllum, Dulcamara, Chamomilla and Bryonia as described earlier in this section, as well as the remedies mentioned below. If none of these remedies is indicated or if well-indicated remedies fail to help, whether the problem is colic, diarrhoea or other digestive disturbances, you should consult a professional homoeopath. You should always do this anyway if symptoms persist, because there are a great many remedies to choose from as well as the possibility of other indications or complications to consider. For instance, small babies may find it hard to digest milk, or may develop digestive symptoms at the time they are weaned; someone could be allergic to a particular food, E number or other additive, and there are numerous other conditions as well, whatever the age of the sufferer, which a professional homoeopath should deal with.

Mag. Phos.

Mag. Phos. pains are always better for pressure, very much better for warmth particularly, and better for rubbing. So with colic, warm drinks will always help, as will a warm hand or hot-water bottle placed on the abdomen. They want to bend double and babies tend to bring their knees up. The pains are cramping and darting in nature. Arsen. Album also is better for warmth but those pains are burning rather than cramping as with Mag. Phos. Chamomilla's colic pains are better for warmth as well but Chamomilla is extremely angry while Mag. Phos. is nervous, tense and twitchy. This remedy always works best if it is dissolved in a little warm water.

Cocculus

The colic pains feel as if the abdomen is full of sharp stones grinding together and there is a lot of distension. Symptoms are accompanied by great weakness particularly of the back and neck. The sufferer generally is worse for cold, better lying quietly on one side, very sensitive to noise and is worse for being jarred, motion and touch.

Colocynth

The most important symptom for this colic is that the pain is better for bending double or for very hard pressure; they want to press something hard against the abdomen for relief and with some people you find them bent over the back of an upright chair or edge of a table in order to get relief. Pains are also better for warmth but pressure relieves the symptoms a great deal more. This is the opposite way round to Mag. Phos. where the colic is mainly better for warmth and to a lesser extent better for pressure. Mentally they have suppressed anger or indignation; this is often hard to discern, particularly with small babies but babies can also get these symptoms if the mother is suppressing anger, vexation, indignation or chagrin. Chamomilla also has colic symptoms coming on with anger, but Colocynth's symptoms are much more from suppressing the emotion.

29. Teething, toothache and gum abscesses

TEETHING

There are three main first aid remedies to choose from for this problem. If your baby does not respond to one of these remedies, or if the teeth are slow or late in appearing, you should consult a homoeopath as it means deeper constitutional treatment is required to prevent suffering.

Chamomilla

This remedy is usually for a very angry baby; angry with the pain of the emerging tooth. The pain is worse for hot drinks and better for cold; your baby will invariably be much crosser after a warm drink than a cool one. Chamomilla babies may well have one cheek red and the other cheek pale, particularly when the double teeth are coming. They may be hot on one side and cold on the other if they are running a temperature, or else their front is cold and their back hot, or vice versa. They are always better for being carried and walked up and down; they calm down and stop yelling if you do this, but begin again at once if you attempt to put them down. Sometimes they may arch their back and throw themselves around in their anger. You would never give this remedy to a quiet, calm baby; they are always irritable to some degree. There may also be colic and diarrhoea with the teething, if so check Chamomilla in section 28. Start with Chamomilla 6 if they are just grizzly cross but go up to a 30 immediately (which may need to be plussed later on) if they get really cross. I nearly always need to start with a 30 when prescribing this remedy and quite frequently a 200 is needed. The remedy works within a few minutes and parents get a peaceful night.

Mag. Phos.

This remedy is the opposite to Chamomilla in that the baby is better for warm drinks and worse for cold drinks. While they may well cry out with the pain of teething they are not angry or irritable but rather twitchy and tense. Start with a 6 and plus it if necessary. This remedy works very well if you dissolve it in a little warm water. You may need to go up to a 30.

Podophyllum

Consider this remedy when the baby is constantly pressing the gums together during teething. There are often profuse and offensive stools during teething (see Podophyllum in section 28).

COLIC AND/OR DIARRHOEA DURING TEETHING

The most likely remedies to be indicated for this are Chamomilla, Podophyllum and Ipecac. You should read section 28 on 'Digestive problems' to get a full picture of the digestive aspects of the three remedies.

TOOTHACHE AND GUM ABSCESSES

If anyone in your family is prone to getting abscesses or mouth ulcers it indicates that they are in need of deeper constitutional treatment; mouth ulcers, for instance, are often indicative of digestive disorders. In these cases please consult a professional homoeopath. Also do not forget to visit your dentist if someone is often getting problems with a particular tooth. It may need treatment or to be removed.

Arnica

This remedy is very useful for any bruising from an injury to the teeth or gums and prevents any long-term damage. Take Arnica 6 three to four times a day for a day or two, stopping as soon as the pain goes. It is useful if your children have general discomfort, aches or bruising, while they are getting accustomed to wearing a plate to straighten their teeth, as well as for adults with new dentures. You can also use this remedy if a tooth needs to be removed as it will reduce any pain from bruising and also prevents excessive bleeding. (See Arnica in section 21 on 'Surgery and operations'.) Calendula Ø undiluted is also excellent in stopping bleeding after a tooth has been removed.

Hypericum

Use this remedy for very sensitive nerve pain and/or nerve injury; pains are worse for touch, cold and pressure. It is useful for any nerve pain when getting used to wearing a plate or dentures. It is also very helpful for the phantom pain which can occur after having a tooth removed. You may need to go up to a 200 or higher, particularly for phantom pain.

Ledum

This remedy is very helpful if you find there is severe pain from an injection in the mouth. (See Ledum in section 15 on 'Punctured wounds'.) A 30 is usually needed here.

Pyrogen

Use this remedy when there is pain from an infected tooth or gum abscess. There is a foul smell from the affected area. Pains are better for warmth and warm drinks. There is a foul taste in the mouth. Start with a 30 and the pain should go very quickly.

Belladonna

Use this remedy in the very earliest stages of a gum abscess, *before* there is any pus, when the area is very red, swollen, throbbing, worse for touch, and worse for cold.

Hepar Sulph.

Use this remedy for gum abscesses before pus has formed or in the early stages once pus has formed. There is extreme sensitivity to touch, cold and air; there are throbbing, pricking pains, the abscess is very inflamed, hot and swollen, pus is scanty but smells like old cheese. Mentally Hepar types are irritable, hasty and vehement. They are generally better in wet weather. Often a 30 or higher will be required. There should be almost immediate relief from pain, followed by re-absorption or discharge of pus and then the swelling goes down.

Silica

Use this remedy for gum abscesses once pus has formed. Pains are burning, cutting, and pulsating, but however extreme the pain, Silica is not particularly worse for touch. Mentally Silica is not the least bit aggressive or angry like Hepar, but much milder, possibly timid or lacking in self-confidence, although very obstinate. Generally they are worse in wet weather and better in warm dry weather. Start the Silica in a 30 or higher and the pus will discharge or be reabsorbed very quickly. **Important note: Do not give this remedy to anyone who has had a transplant of any kind, or a pacemaker, or has shrapnel from old war wounds or other injuries; it is just possible that Silica could try to push these out too.**

30. Headaches

It is very important to realize that if there is a tendency to get headaches fairly often they are nearly always part of a deeper chronic condition affecting the whole person (and which could very occasionally indicate serious pathology). Headaches which are part of a chronic condition are often connected with digestive problems of many kinds including constipation; they may well follow head injuries; they may result from using ointments to suppress some scalp condition or from using the conventional medications to treat head lice. They may be associated with sinus or catarrhal problems, particularly suppressing these with ordinary medicines; for women, they may be associated with menstruation or the menopause. These are just a few examples of the numerous chronic conditions which may be associated with headaches, for which professional homoeopathic treatment should be sought. This should reduce the tendency to get frequent acute headaches and should also avoid any serious underlying condition developing. For treating acute headaches yourself there are a vast number of remedies to choose from so I have included only those which get used very frequently. You should also bear in mind that acute headaches often accompany many of the acute childhood diseases, as well as fevers, colds and earaches. If this is the case the appropriate section on these ailments should be read in conjunction with this section.

Aconite

These headaches are violent and throbbing with sudden onset, like Belladonna. Pains may be worse around 9 pm or in the night, worse in a warm room, better in open air and better for uncovering. There may be a sensation of a hot band surrounding the head and the head itself will be hot and burning. There is thirst for cool things. Mentally Aconite is extremely fearful, anxious and restless. As always with Aconite, it is needed in the early stages and the symptoms may come on from exposure to cold dry windy weather, or after a fright of some kind. It is useful for headaches which accompany the early stages of colds, fevers, coughs, earache, and the acute childhood diseases, so refer to these sections in this book.

Actea Rac. (also known as Cimicifuga)

This headache remedy is indicated when the pains are pressing outwards particularly; the brain feels too big for the head and it feels as if the top of the head will fly off; or the pressure can go into the eyes making them ache, or go to the neck with shooting pains towards the spine. Sufferers feel better for keeping warm but like open air too, and are twitchy, nauseous, trembling, and gloomy.

Belladonna

The onset of the Belladonna headache is fast and it can disappear equally quickly. They are always better sitting up propped against pillows rather than lying down flat. The head is usually better for leaning it gently against something, worse for touch and the scalp is very sensitive. They want the doors and windows shut as they feel worse for draughts. Light hurts their eyes so that they want the room darkened and curtains drawn; the pupils of the eyes are usually dilated. The actual pains are throbbing and pulsating, often coming in waves. The face is usually red and hot. Belladonna headaches often start around 3 pm or 3 am, or become worse at these times. There is thirst usually for cold water or lemonade. The pain is worse for motion, may well be worse on the right side and is sometimes better actually bending the head back. There are many things which can bring on this kind of headache but in particular hot sun (see section 31 on 'Sunstroke'), as well as exposure to cold wet weather, and washing or cutting the hair. It is a headache which often accompanies fevers, coughs, colds and sore throats, as well as the acute childhood diseases, so you may need to refer to the appropriate sections in this book. Mentally they can be restless, irritable, grumpy, or really quarrelsome.

Bryonia

These headaches are always very much worse for the slightest movement or jar and better for hard pressure; sufferers are, however, extremely irritated by light touch. If you see the patient sitting as still as possible holding his head firmly, you should consider this remedy. There is thirst for large quantities at a time. The pain can be crushing, stitching, heavy or splitting. It is a headache which can come on from cooling down suddenly when overheated. This headache can accompany fevers, coughs, colds, constipation, and the acute childhood diseases, (particularly if a rash has been slow to emerge or has been suppressed).

Gelsemium

This headache often comes on after exposure to hot sun (see section 31 on 'Sunstroke') and also may accompany fevers, colds, and the acute childhood diseases, (see those sections). They are usually trembling or shaky and feel extraordinarily weak. The pain is usually worse at the base of the head at the back. There is generally no thirst and as the headache begins to improve there is an increase in urination. The most comfortable position is to sit propped with the head upright; the face is pale, or occasionally dusky red. The pains can be preceded by visual disturbances as in migraine, which improve as the headache gets worse. Please do not assume that this is the only remedy for migraine – there are hundreds to choose from and the *remedy must fit the totality of the picture presented by the patient* in order to be homoeopathic and to result in a cure. (You should consult a professional homoeopath for treating migraine.)

Kali Bich.

This is a remedy which is particularly indicated for catarrhal and sinus type headaches as is Pulsatilla. The distinguishing feature with Kali Bich. is that the pain is very sharp and penetrating but covers a small area that can be covered with the tip of one's finger. It is similar to Gelsemium in that there can be visual disturbances at the beginning which improve as the headache gets worse. Kali Bich. headaches are better for warmth and for pressure.

Nux Vomica

This is an excellent remedy for the typical hangover headache and the headache that often accompanies overeating, drinking too much alcohol, diarrhoea, and colds. The head feels enlarged, the scalp is very sensitive, and Nux Vomica types feel better leaning the head against something (Belladonna). Pains can be bruising, splitting, digging, or squeezing and patients are better keeping still, lying down, covered up and in a warm room; they are worse for noise and there is a bruised kind of sensation. Mentally they are intensely irritable and over-sensitive.

Phosphorus

Although Phosphorus is generally better for warmth and worse for cold their headaches are in fact worse for heat and better for cold. They are also worse for noise, light, lying and motion, and better sitting, eating, and for sleep. They may describe a peculiar feeling of bubbles coming up the back of the head. Generally they are worse at dusk. They are restless all over although the headache itself is worse for motion. It is one of the remedies particularly indicated for children who have been growing fast and also for hunger headaches when there is pain over one eye as well. Phosphorus types are worse alone, outgoing, always enjoy people and company and are very demonstrative.

Pulsatilla

Pulsatilla type headaches may occur particularly when accompanying mumps, measles, rubella, the digestive symptoms from overeating rich food, or else from sinus and catarrhal congestion following a cold (see those sections). They are seldom thirsty, better in open air and worse for warm rooms, worse in the evenings, better for company and attention, better lying with the head propped high or better when walking gently around. Symptoms may change a lot, both the type of pain as well as the location of the pain.

31. Sunstroke

There are three main remedies to consider for sunstroke although it is much better to prevent your family from getting it in the first place, particularly as we are now also aware of the dangers of skin cancer from overexposure to the sun. (You should use Urtica or Cantharis, see section 19 on 'Burns', if you need to treat sunburn. Usually Urtica will be all you need but for extremely severe sunburn with blisters you should use Cantharis.) For sunstroke you will find that Belladonna, Glonoine or Gelsemium will help.

The main symptoms of sunstroke are that the temperature rises to

39°C (or frequently higher), sweating ceases, there is dizziness, nausea, weakness and headache, and in severe cases it can lead to confusion, delirium and coma. There can also be vomiting, convulsions, raised blood pressure, fast pulse and rapid breathing.

Belladonna

There is a pulsating, throbbing, bursting headache. Sufferers are worse lying flat and better sitting propped up; the giddiness and headache are worse when stooping and from motion; they are worse for touch and worse for uncovering and draughts (opposite to Glonoine); pupils are dilated, the face hot and red with dry skin. Also Belladonna is often better bending the head backwards and the pain may appear to surge up and down. Severe cases can have delirium and loss of consciousness, twitching, spasms and convulsions. If there is delirium and the sufferer is being 'energetic' with it, start with Belladonna 30 plussing it if necessary; you may need to go up to a 200; otherwise start with Belladonna 6 which may well be all that is needed.

Glonoine

There is a bursting, throbbing, pounding headache; the pain comes in waves with an expanding and contracting sensation, or as if surging backwards and forwards. They are better sitting propped up, worse for motion, worse for sun and worse for touch. The face is red or possibly bluish, but can be pale if there is vomiting which relieves the nausea. Unlike Belladonna they are better in open air and for uncovering as well as being worse when bending the head backwards. They just sit holding their head as still as possible with their elbows on their knees. There are palpitations and pulsations throughout the whole body.

Gelsemium

Gelsemium symptoms are much less violent than either Belladonna or Glonoine. The fever is not so high and there is little if any throbbing. They are better for sitting propped with the head high and better for urination. There can be a lot of trembling, shaking and great weakness. The face is pale or dusky red, not bright red like Belladonna or bluish red like Glonoine. They are usually thirstless.

32. Exam anticipation nerves

The remedies mentioned in this chapter are only for *temporary* anticipatory fears; such as when children have important tests or examinations at school, as well as before some performance such as acting in a school play or making an announcement during assembly. Adults find these remedies useful if they are nervous before making speeches, important meetings, interviews, as well as examinations. You should consult a professional homoeopath for treatment of *long-term* anxieties, anticipation and fearfulness. Homoeopathy can help enormously with these kinds of conditions; it can not only dramatically improve the happiness and future development of children with such problems, but also prevent these types of anxieties from ruining career or promotion prospects for adults.

Gelsemium

Use this remedy for temporary anticipatory fears such as those before an exam or some kind of performance. Symptoms for this remedy are predominantly shaking, trembling and lack of muscular co-ordination; their legs shake so much they can hardly stand up. Writing is poor because their hands are trembling. Their mind goes blank and all knowledge their seems to be lost. If you are certain that a remedy will be required it is best to take a dose on rising on the morning of the exam or performance and another dose immediately before it. Usually there should be no need for another dose during the exam, unless symptoms persist.

Use the remedy in a 12 first; occasionally you may need to go up to a 30.

Argent. Nit.

This remedy, again only for *temporary* anticipation nerves, is indicated when the main symptoms are an increase in urination and/or diarrhoea prior to an exam. There can be trembling as well, but the emphasis is on the increased frequency of urination or diarrhoea. They are overexcitable and again the mind goes blank so that they cannot remember what they have learned. Follow the same potency instructions as for Gelsemium above.

Rescue Remedy with Mimulus

This is a combination of the Bach remedies and is best used as a liquid remedy. It does not come in a potency. Rescue Remedy helps with the general panic and fear, while Mimulus helps with fear of a known specific thing; this mixture is probably most useful if you feel the symptoms do not fit either Gelsemium or Argent. Nit.

Take two to three drops, preferably in a little water, three times a day starting a few days before the occasion. It can then be taken as frequently as required on the day concerned. However, I think it is best to forget about the remedy during an exam; only taking it (direct onto the tongue during an actual exam as that is simplest) if symptoms are particularly bad, which should be unlikely by then.

33. Conjunctivitis

This is when the mucous membrane which lines the eyelids and eyeball becomes inflamed and sore. There is usually redness of the whites of the eye, lachrymation and often a thick discharge as well as soreness and pain. Conjunctivitis can accompany some of the childhood diseases, particularly mumps, measles and rubella, see chapter four. If you get conjunctivitis frequently then it is important to consult a homoeopath in order to have treatment for the chronic condition which will prevent you getting it in the first place.

Argent. Nit.

Use this remedy when there is a very profuse thick bland discharge which can be creamy in colour, greenish-yellow, green or yellow. The whites of the eye may be red or pink and may actually be swollen. They are better for cool air and cool bathing of the eye.

Pulsatilla

This remedy also has a thick bland discharge which is green, yellow, cream, or greenish yellow. It is not quite so profuse as the Argent. Nit. discharge but there is still a lot of it. One keynote is that the colour changes between green, yellow, and cream. The eyes itch a good deal. The patient's moods change too; one minute they will be laughing, the next they will be crying. The eyes are better for anything cool. The patient thrives on sympathy and attention.

Sulphur

Here there is not very much thick discharge but there is a lot of lachrymation. The rims of the eyes will be very red and look and feel very sore. Like Pulsatilla it will be itchy, and will also be sore and burning. They will be unlikely to want them bathed.

Euphrasia

Here the eyes water all the time with lots of hot burning tears. The discharge is usually thick yellow and acrid (Merc. Sol. is thin and acrid). As well as taking the remedy internally, you can put two drops of Euphrasia Ø into an eyebath of boiled then cooled water; use this to bathe the eye and you will find it a great help. You can do this whichever remedy you are taking.

DOSAGE

With any of the above remedies I would start with a 12 or a 30 and take it three to four times a day for up to about four days at the most. Stop the remedy as soon as there is improvement, but start again should the symptoms return. It should usually clear up in a few days or less. If the conjunctivitis comes on during one of the childhood diseases check in chapter four to make sure that you have chosen the most similar remedy.

34. Worms

The following remedy is suitable for worms known as round worms, thread worms, pin worms or ascarides lumbricoides. Although there is no reason why you should not try treating these yourself, if improvement is only slight or is not lasting then you must seek professional help. This is because the problem is more chronic in nature, and constitutional treatment is required to remove the tendency to being susceptible to them in the first place. As far as tapeworms are concerned I think it is best to consult your homoeopath.

Cina

This is the main remedy to consider for worms. If a patient needs Cina he tends to pick his nose a lot, may grind his teeth during sleep and can be as cross as Chamomilla (see section 29 on 'Teething'). He may alternate between having bright red cheeks and pale face with dark circles round the eyes; or else he could have a red face but with paleness round the mouth and nose. (Chamomilla has one side red and hot and the other side pale.) There can be ravenous hunger one minute and no appetite whatsoever the next. Give Cina 6 three times a day for up to four days, remembering to stop before the four days are up if improvement begins before that (which it often does). Sometimes it may seem that the symptoms are worse but it is simply the body pushing out all the worms; if this is the case use Rescue Remedy cream or Hypercal cream to prevent any soreness, and stop the remedy; it means that enough has been taken to stimulate a cure. Some people prefer to take Cina 200, three doses in one day only and then wait for a few weeks for the remedy to work. The worms should disappear and you only repeat it if symptoms return.

35. Head lice

Over the years it seems that head lice have developed resistance to the usual shampoos and lotions and these medications have had to become much stronger in order to deal with them. I have found that some children find these strong applications give them the most frightful headaches; these can be so painful that you find the children banging their heads against the wall to get relief. Automatic use of these medications is quite unnecessary anyway; people only get the lice if they are susceptible, as with any disease.

There has been research (reported in *The Observer* newspaper on 28 March 1993) by the Chronic Disease Prevention Division at the Missouri Department of Health into the connection between exposure to pesticides and brain cancer. The research concluded that there is a 'significant positive association' between the incidence of childhood brain cancer and exposure to lindane, carbaryl, dichlorvos and diazinon – these are all active ingredients in the insecticides used to control head lice (as well as to control household bugs and garden pests).

Head lice in children can be dealt with by mixing up a lotion of one part Staphisagria Ø to four parts water and leaving this on the scalp to dry naturally. This may have to be repeated frequently at first (possibly as often as once every few days for up to about five occasions) with some children. Please remember that Staphisagria Ø is unpotentised and **should not be drunk**. It is quite safe to use on the scalp when diluted as described above.

The use of hair conditioner, left thickly on the hair for a while after washing, is also a good method to get rid of head lice. Lavender, Bergamot and Geranium aromatherapy oils can also help in this condition. The blend of these oils should be 5–10 parts oil to 95–90 parts carrier oil and left on the scalp for a few hours, or over night, before washing out. Do not use eucalyptus oil or tea tree oil (melaleuca alternifolia oil) as they can antidote your homoeopathic remedies if you are undergoing homoeopathic treatment (see pages 23–25). Helios Homoeopathic Pharmacy (see page 211) now do a Lice Solution. Any of these methods should be combined with the use of a nit comb in order to get a good result. If, despite this the lice return, it means internal homoeopathic treatment is needed as well to stop the susceptibility to getting the lice in the first place; you should therefore consult your homoeopath.

Chapter Four

THE ACUTE CHILDHOOD DISEASES

The following section on the acute childhood diseases should make it much easier for you to decide whether or not to vaccinate your children. It should give you the confidence and the knowledge to treat them yourself, or with the help of a homoeopathic practitioner for the more serious conditions. There is an increased awareness today of the probable long-term damage to the immune system from vaccinations and section 36 touches on some of these disadvantages and dangers, suggesting further reading for parents who want a wider understanding of this subject. Subsequent sections deal with the treatment and prevention for each individual acute childhood disease.

DOSAGE AND POTENCY GENERALLY

Throughout this chapter, unless I have indicated that you should use a specific potency for a particular situation or ailment, please remember to follow the advice given in the section on 'Rules about dosage, potencies and repetition of doses' on pages 30–35.

36. Inoculations and vaccinations

When people first grasp the idea of the law of similars, or of treating like with like as in homoeopathic medicine, they tend to assume that it is the same as vaccination and inoculation. This is in fact not the case at all. When you vaccinate against a particular disease you administer an identical substance to the disease; it has nothing to do with the uniqueness of the individual. Homoeopathy involves giving a substance which though different in nature is similar in expression; you match the symptoms unique to that sick individual to those the remedy can produce in a healthy person. Also with homoeopathy the remedy is given in a potency, that is as an energy, which is gentle and safe, not as a material foreign substance or disease product being pumped straight into the bloodstream. The preservatives and carrier substances for the vaccines which are being sent straight into the bloodstream as well, should also be a cause for anxiety from the toxicity point of view. *The Sunday Times* reported on 3 June 2001 that "The government's medicines safety watchdog has taken action to warn patients and GPs of potential serious adverse reactions to vaccines containing a preservative which is almost 50% mercury". A warning will have to be added to the vaccine summary of product characteristics, and on the patient information leaflet, for vaccines with thiomersal. The vaccines that currently contain thiomersal are the DPT vaccines and the DT vaccines. Apart from thiomersal, which is a mercury derivative, the other ingredients used in vaccines for preservative reasons and which are suspected of causing damage are formaldehyde, aluminium sulphate, phenol, ethylene glycol, benzethonium chloride, and methylparaben. (See *What Doctors Don't Tell You,* volume 12, no 5 for more details about these substances.) Aluminium, mercury and formaldehyde are all substances which can be turned into homoeopathic potencies. In other words they have been made completely safe by the dilution and succussion process so that no single molecule of the original substance is left, and only an energy pattern, unique to that substance, remains. Homoeopaths use them as remedies, **but only *after* they have been diluted and succussed until there is nothing of the original poison left in them.** They are used during homoeopathic treatment for many conditions when patients present symptom pictures similar to the poisonous effects of those substances. That means they are used for symptoms which are similar to the drug pictures or provings of these substances. For this reason homoeopaths know exactly what damage these substances can cause to the body in very great detail. Anyone who wants to know what side effects these substances can cause only has to look them up in a good homoeopathic *Materia Medica* and read the remedy provings. Like all homoeopathic remedies made from originally poisonous substances, there is nothing left in the remedy of the original poison, and only a unique energy remains. Remedies made from them either do absolutely nothing, if given to someone who is *not* presenting similar symptoms, but cure the symptoms if given to someone who *is* presenting similar symptoms. Since we know in such detail the symptoms these preservative substances could cause, we should be even more concerned about potential vaccine damage; not only from the disease products themselves but from the preservatives as well. (See also Appendix 4.)

I am not going to go into the pros and cons of vaccinations in any depth in this book. There are four excellent books on the subject which every parent should read before they subject their children to vaccination. One is *Mass Immunisation*, a fairly short booklet of some thirty pages, by Trevor Gunn (ISBN 0 9517657 1 X), published by Cutting Edge Publications; another is *Vaccination and Immunization* by Leon Chaitow (ISBN 0 85207 191 4), published by C.W. Daniel Company Ltd; the third is *DPT, A Shot in the Dark* by Harris L. Coulter and Barbara Fisher (ISBN 0 15 126481 3) published by Harcourt Brace Jovanovich, 1985 and the fourth is a booklet called *The WDDTY Vaccination Handbook*, available from Satellite House, 2 Salisbury Road, London SW19 4EZ. Telephone 020-8944-9555. This last one concentrates mostly on the short-term rather than long-term damage, as well as the actual long-term ineffectiveness of the vaccinations; the other three cover much wider aspects, including possible long-term harm manifesting itself later on in life.

There is now evidence to show that the statistical claims that immunization has helped in the elimination of these diseases are inaccurate; the incidence of the diseases was already declining dramatically by the time immunization programmes began and the statistics merely show a continuation of those decreasing numbers. At the same time there have been reforms in public health which have led to cleaner water, decent sanitation, better housing and better diets. These reforms have increased people's resistance to the diseases and decreased the severity and virulence along with the numbers of cases. Scarlet fever, for which a vaccine was never developed, began to decrease of its own accord and has now virtually died out. There is every reason to suppose, since this had already begun to happen in significant numbers with the other diseases prior to the introduction of the vaccination programmes, that they would have gradually died out as well. The fact that the incidence of some of these diseases gets lower year by year is just as likely, if not more likely, to be due to the natural waning of the diseases and increased *natural* immunity, as in scarlet fever, than to the vaccinations. If people find this hard to credit, they should consider the fact that over and over again Leon Chaitow and others quote reliable statistics which demonstrate that the incidence of these diseases has been as high, and sometimes higher, in groups of people who have been immunized than in those who have not been immunized. The fact that these vaccines only seem to provide a temporary immunity is particularly worrying as all these illnesses are much more serious if caught when an adult.

There is also evidence to show that in the long-term immunization weakens the immune system (by keeping it in a constant state of alertness ready to fight off these diseases), and is one of the causes of the increasing incidence of auto-immune diseases. This occurs when the body produces antibodies against normal healthy parts of the body to such an extent as to cause tissue injury, such as in multiple sclerosis, cancer, rheumatoid arthritis and diabetes. Various kinds of central nervous system dysfunction, accompanied or followed by serious disruptive, violent and antisocial behaviour, have also been associated with immunization damage – and all of these serious chronic conditions are dramatically on the increase. While there may well be many contributing factors for the increase in violence of all kinds in recent years there is no reason to suppose that widespread immunization has not played a part. When an acute disease such as scarlet fever is not suppressed and is able to die out naturally, it is because natural immunity has been acquired and because the disease is no longer necessary to throw off particular miasmatic weaknesses or to strengthen the vitality. It appears that immunization against the other acute childhood diseases has prevented the natural outlet of the vital force from trying to push diseases out to the periphery, instead driving diseases inwards only to mutate into more dangerous forms. It is now also thought to be highly likely that the enormous rise in numbers in recent years of less serious but nevertheless chronic conditions is mostly attributable to vaccination side effects; depending on the inoculation, these conditions include breathing difficulties and asthma, eczema, anorexia and bulimia, allergies, colic, dyslexia, glue ear, lowered resistance to infection, sterility, temper tantrums, hyperactivity and tendencies to addiction, to mention only a few.

When probable cause and effect are separated by months or, more usually, by years, there is no reason to ignore or scoff at such a possibility just because it is less obvious and less easy to prove. Why on earth increase the risk of debilitating, painful and serious chronic disease later on in life as a consequence of vaccination, simply in order to avoid childhood diseases which can be so easily and successfully treated with homoeopathy? If health can be increased by proper cleanliness and a good diet, and if homoeopathic remedies are used to treat the childhood diseases themselves, why damage the immune system by an unnecessary vaccination with all the possible risks attached; not just the devastating consequences which occasionally happen almost immediately after an injection, but the deep-seated, long-term, chronic diseases of the damaged immune system? If you are in two minds about this I beg you to read the books I have mentioned.

On the whole vaccinations have had a very good press for a long time but as always only a small and extremely misleading part of the story has been told. We have been bombarded with literature emphasizing the dangers of the diseases so that we react with our emotions, in this case the fear of the diseases, and we have been given very little information on the potential dangers of immunization. There have been various bonus payments made to doctors for giving vaccinations which encourage them to vaccinate as many children as possible. These financial incentives lead to an enormous amount of pressure being put onto parents to have their children vaccinated, which can be hard to resist. Parents are encouraged to fear the possible seriousness of the diseases if they are left untreated, and are made to feel extremely guilty about the possibility of infecting other people.

You should not let this sway you because if their vaccines really worked then they should not need to be worried about infection. By using homoeopathic remedies you should find that the diseases themselves should be extremely mild; your children should also obtain lifelong immunity from the diseases once they have had them, which is not the case from the inoculations. (You should of course be very careful about the dangers of spreading infection with rubella, see section 41.)

From an economic point of view it is much simpler and cheaper in the short-term for governments to run vaccination programmes than to concentrate on improving nutrition, cleanliness and the availability of clean water. Is this the reason why only one very distorted part of the story has ever been publicized, or are the so-called experts advising governments so blinkered that they cannot see what has really happened? Much literature (or rather propaganda as it relies on people's ignorance) which stirs up people's fears and also ridicules any other differing points of view, has contributed to preventing the truth from being aired. As said before there has been a vast increase in serious chronic diseases dating back to the introduction of vaccinations. To some extent this must have resulted from the mass immunization programmes suppressing natural disease outlets and causing their mutation into far more serious diseases. This must in part have contributed to the ever rising costs of the National Health Service which we see today in Great Britain. Even if one looks only at the economics of the situation, but from a long-term point of view, this surely must be an argument for a radical change of policy and direction.

There are real advantages in actually having the acute childhood diseases because they enable people to rid themselves to some extent of the miasmatic weaknesses (see page 7) which we all inherit. These weaknesses lead to increased tendencies to succumb to serious chronic diseases later in life. Professional homoeopaths are perfectly capable of treating all the childhood diseases with minimum fuss and suffering for the patient. There is no reason why any of these diseases should become serious if homoeopathic treatment is given and the patient is generally well cared for. The two main benefits from having had the childhood diseases are (1) that you obtain genuine lifelong immunity and (2) the whole long-term future health of people (and their descendants) will be much improved and strengthened, reducing susceptibility to serious chronic diseases later on, since many miasmatic weakness will have been thrown off. As homoeopaths we are constantly treating people with serious debilitating chronic diseases. It really is exasperating as well as desperately sad to know that if the vaccinations and suppressions our patients have experienced earlier in their lives had been avoided, then much of their present suffering would either never have happened, or would have been much less severe.

Luckily in England we are still free to choose and this chapter gives you the chance to use homoeopathic remedies as an alternative if you wish to do so. I have tried to make the advice as simple and as comprehensive as possible. It is in the Third World where there are poor standards of hygiene and cleanliness, diet is frequently inadequate and clean water hard to find, that the acute childhood diseases are often very serious. It is important to understand that a good diet, cleanliness, plenty of fresh air and exercise help build up health and strength in your children, thereby reducing the severity of these diseases. With homoeopathic treatment as well during the acute illness, as described in the following sections, there is no reason why these illnesses should become prolonged or develop into more serious conditions. These diseases should tend to be so mild and the suffering so slight that you will wonder what all the fuss was about. It is anyway considered to be much more satisfactory to catch these illnesses during childhood as this is the best way to get genuine lifelong immunity. You will also be giving your children a much better start in life without running the risk of them succumbing to the more long-term serious consequences of inoculations, as well as helping them throw off some of the miasmatic weaknesses which we all inherit. I suggest you contact your local homoeopath for support; they will be pleased to know what you are up to and will give you professional advice.

37. Chickenpox

It is important to be able to differentiate between chickenpox and smallpox (despite the fact that smallpox is thought to have been eradicated) as smallpox can be misdiagnosed as chickenpox. The chief difference is that with chickenpox the spots are all at different stages of development; with some small clear blisters or vesicles and others much larger, as well as scabs and crusts. This is because new spots appear every few days whereas in smallpox the spots are all at the same stage, that is they are all blisters, or all scabby crusts. The chickenpox spots are much softer to touch than the smallpox ones which are deeper and hard. The other way to differentiate is by the location of the spots. Chickenpox spots are most thick on the chest and back and spread less thickly to the face, upper arms and upper legs. Smallpox spots are mostly on the face and scalp rather than the trunk and more on the lower arms, hands and wrists, lower legs and feet, rather than the upper arms and thighs. Smallpox is also preceded by severe backache and prostration for three to four days before there is any eruption.

The incubation period for chickenpox is two to three weeks. The rash starts with flat spots which become raised and then turn into vesicles, or small blisters, containing clear fluid. These in turn become pustules within about 48 hours. The spots itch, become dry and form scabs or crusts which eventually heal up and fall off. It can be caught from contact with chickenpox blisters and from shingles blisters as well as from droplet infection. The skin eruptions are usually accompanied by a slight fever, headache and generally aching limbs.

Do not put any lotions on the spots as it is quite likely that a lotion will upset the curative action of the homoeopathic remedy. Do not give any remedies together. It should always be clear which is the most indicated remedy at any given time.

Antim. Tart.

This is of most use during the early stages, particularly if the rash is slow to develop. It is especially indicated if the patient has a cough or bronchitis along with the rash or before the rash comes out properly.

The cough is loose with a lot of rattling mucus in the lungs. Patients are irritable and worse for heat and covering.

Start with Antim. Tart. 6, three or four times a day for a few days, remembering to adjust the frequency according to any improvement; only a few doses may be required. Remember that as the cough improves the rash should come out more; this is very important as it demonstrates that the disease is going from within outwards, i.e. from a more serious part (lungs) to a less serious part (skin).

Rhus Tox.

This remedy is most used when the itching from the rash is bad and there is a lot of restlessness. There is no need to put on any lotions to stop the itching because this remedy will not only stop the itch but will speed up the healing and disappearance of the eruptions. You should always deal with the cough first (if there is one) by giving Antim. Tart. and only then go onto Rhus Tox. to heal the rash. Start with Rhus Tox. 6 as often as required, taking it whenever the itch is bad.

Merc. Sol.

This remedy is indicated when there are internal painful, pustular spots such as in the mouth (like mouth ulcers) or in the eyes or nose; the breath is smelly and the spots externally are larger, more painful and pustular. There is usually a lot of sweating which does not bring relief, and they are worse at night and fairly weak. Such symptoms are more likely in the more severe cases which tend to occur in older children or adults. Merc. Sol. 30 is the best potency to start with here. I have seldom found that I have needed more than six doses during a 24–48 hour period.

Sulphur

Sometimes you may need to give Sulphur 6 twice a day for a few days if the sufferer seems to be tired, weak and not picking up properly once the disease is over.

PREVENTION

You can give Varicella 30 morning and evening on one day then once a week for three more doses if there has been contact with the disease or if there is an outbreak locally. However, this is such a mild disease when treated with homoeopathic remedies that there seems very little point in specific prevention.

38. Smallpox

Please see the first paragraph of the previous section on chickenpox so that you can differentiate between smallpox and chickenpox. For both prevention and treatment of smallpox the best remedy is Variolinum.

In the unlikely event that you are travelling to an area where there is still thought to be a risk of smallpox, give Variolinum 30 night and morning on one day initially, then one dose every fourth day for three more doses. Thereafter give one dose once every two weeks until the danger is over.

For the actual disease, give Variolinum 30 night and morning, stopping as soon as there is improvement, and repeating if symptoms relapse. The illness should be very mild and short lasting and pitting should be prevented. As smallpox is now considered to have been eradicated there seems little point in going into further details of the numerous other remedies which can be indicated for treating it; also the treatment and prevention outlined in this chapter should be very effective. As with any serious disease you should seek professional homoeopathic advice if necessary.

39. Mumps

Known side effects (of the more immediate kind) of the MMR (measles, mumps and rubella) vaccine, are encephalitis, seizure, meningitis and deafness. Latterly autism, digestive problems and Crohn's disease have also been attributed to it. Statistics vary as to the likelihood of such risks, but put into the context of (a) the disease being considered only a very mild illness when treated homoeopathically, (b) the short-term and imperfect immunity obtained from the vaccination and (c) the miasmatic weaknesses which will be reduced by having had mumps itself, such serious risks simply cannot be worth it. Also do not forget about the long-term damage to the immune system from the vaccination and the risks of more serious disease much later on (see section 36). Homoeopathic treatment for mumps is straightforward and any suffering should be very slight.

The incubation period is about three weeks and the early symptoms are those of a slightly feverish cold with a temperature of about 39°C and a runny nose. There will be tenderness around the ears, usually only on one side, followed by the swelling of the parotid gland. This gland lies all round the ear lobe, that is in front, below and behind it; it is hard and immovable. (In other illnesses where glands in this area are swollen they are movable.) With the swelling of the parotid gland the shape of the face changes completely giving a somewhat absurd appearance. There is pain when eating and even when opening the mouth because the parotid duct (which is inside the mouth and looks like a red dot between the upper and lower molars) usually gets swollen. Saliva is usually increased considerably. The parotid gland can be swollen on either one or both sides of the face. The patient is infectious for seven days after the first swollen gland appears or until the glands recede. Complications which can follow are orchitis, which is inflammation of the testicles, inflammation of the ovaries, mastitis, or meningitis. These complications should be preventable with homoeopathic treatment; if necessary seek professional homoeopathic advice.

Pilocarpine

This remedy covers all the usual mumps symptoms described above. Start with Pilocarpine 6 at least twice a day until the symptoms have gone; make sure you follow the instructions in section 10 about 'Dosage, potencies and repetition of doses'. The disease should last only a few days and improvement should begin after the first dose.

Pilocarpine should prevent it becoming serious, prevent the onset of complications and cut short the disease. (The remedy Jaborandi has also been used with as much success – Pilocarpine is an alkaloid which has been isolated from the Jaborandi tree.)

Merc. Sol.

Occasionally this remedy is more indicated than Pilocarpine. The chief symptoms are very smelly breath with a heavily coated tongue, heavy sweats which do not relieve and exhaustion. You would never consider giving Merc. Sol. unless there was the very smelly breath. It is often worse on the right side. It is also indicated if there is either mastitis or orchitis along with the other Merc. Sol. modalities. Give Merc. Sol. 30 as often as necessary till these symptoms have gone; it is unlikely that the remedy will be needed for more than a few days. If the Merc. Sol. symptoms disappear leaving just the usual mumps symptoms, it is occasionally necessary to follow it with Pilocarpine 6.

Parotidinum Nosode 30

Although I have always used Pilocarpine 6 in preference to this remedy, it is supposed to be just as good. It can be used night and morning from when the symptoms begin and the illness usually clears up quickly with no complications.

Belladonna

This is for bright red shiny swelling on the right side only, or worse on the right side; also for great thirst and sensitivity to light, noise and draughts, and worse around 3 pm or 3 am. With mastitis there are red streaks radiating from the centre plus the other Belladonna modalities.

Bryonia

Use this for very dry lips and mouth, with great thirst, irritability and general aggravation from motion; also relief from cool air and aggravation from light touch. There is mastitis with stony hard breasts along with the other Bryonia modalities.

Lycopodium

This is for swelling which begins on the right side and may move to the left; better for warm drinks and generally worse around 4 pm.

Lachesis

Use this for swelling which is worse on the left side and may cross over to the right side; the throat and the swollen glands are worse for any sort of touch or pressure, even the touch of clothing. They are better for cool drinks. Give it for mastitis if the breasts are bluish and inflamed along with the other Lachesis modalities.

Rhus Tox.

This is used if the swelling is dark red and on the left side; also with thirst for milk, sensitivity to draughts and restlessness. It is also indicated if swelling of testes remains following mumps, providing there are the other Rhus Tox. modalities as well.

Pulsatilla

Pulsatilla is indicated for thirstlessness, craving for fresh air and aggravation from overheating. Their mood is usually tearful and/or changeable, and they are worse when alone. Use it if there is mastitis or orchitis along with these modalities.

Phytolacca

Pains shoot into the ear when swallowing and the parotid gland is stony hard. This is also indicated for stony hard breasts in mastitis with pain spreading from them all over the body. Symptoms are worse in cold and wet weather.

PREVENTION

There are a variety of ways to approach this but one of the following should suit you:

a) You could give Parotidinum 30, one dose a year for a very young child up to the age of about three, starting from the date the child would normally be given its first MMR inoculation. After this age it is much better to get the illness and treat it as described above or follow the advice in b) below.

b) Once you become aware of an outbreak of mumps in the neighbourhood you could give Parotidinum 30 twice (morning and evening) on one day initially then once every fourth day after that for three more doses; thereafter the dose is once every ten to fourteen days until the danger is over. If mumps actually developed the case should be very mild and easily treatable, usually with Pilocarpine or possibly one of the other remedies described in this chapter.

c) You could do a) as well as b) above.

Personally I would not bother with any prevention unless a child is very young or for a person who is not very strong, and then I would do b) above. Otherwise I would simply use homoeopathic treatment once the illness had developed, so as to obtain lifelong immunity.

40. Measles

As with most complications from the childhood diseases, statistics on measles show that these occur almost exclusively among extremely low income families where it is hard to avoid very poor nutrition, inadequate living conditions and poor hygiene; but if you are able to feed and take care of your children sensibly and well, the possiblility of complications should be reduced. Also, there has been evidence to show that the measles part of the MMR vaccine does not appear to work for long. Outbreaks of the disease in the late 1980s demonstrated that over two thirds of the cases occurred in children who *had* been vaccinated.

THE ACUTE CHILDHOOD DISEASES

There is also the risk of vaccination damaging the immune system, resulting in auto-immune diseases later on in life (see section 36).

The early symptoms of measles are similar to a feverish cold – a raised temperature, a runny nose, catarrh and a cough. The only particular indication for measles at this stage is that there are little white flecks or spots, known as Koplik's spots, inside the cheeks opposite the molars. A few days later the fever rises and a rash appears first behind the ears and spreading to the face and chest; as the rash appears the Koplik's spots usually disappear. The rash, consisting of pinkish slightly raised blotches which soon run into each other, lasts about seven days. The rash has clearly defined edges (unlike scarlet fever where the rash fades gradually at the edges). Accompanying symptoms can be conjunctivitis and photophobia, mild bronchitis and otitis media. You should also check in the other sections of this book if any of these symptoms accompany the measles symptoms; ('Fevers', section 23, 'Earache', section 25, 'Coughs', section 27 and 'Conjunctivitis', section 33). This should help in the remedy choices. With homoeopathic treatment none of these symptoms should become serious and the illness should only last a short time; if necessary you should seek professional homoeopathic advice.

Aconite

This remedy is indicated most frequently for normally strong, healthy children with rosy cheeks. The onset is sudden with great restlessness, burning heat and thirst. They are extremely anxious and agitated and usually frightened. The eyes may seem glassy with the pupils contracted. They may well have been exposed to cold, dry windy weather earlier that day. If there is a cough it will be dry, hacking and croupy. There can be vomiting and diarrhoea. They may be worse at about 9 pm. and will throw off the bedclothes, not wanting to be covered up.

Start with Aconite 6 unless there is a great deal of restlessness and anxiety, in which case start with a 30. If the fever is very high, remember you may need to give the remedy quite often initially as it will be 'burnt up' more quickly.

Antim. Crud.

This remedy is for those who are peevish and cross. The face is hot and red like Aconite and Belladonna but there is no thirst or anxiety. The corners of the mouth are sore and cracked, sometimes the nostrils are cracked as well and the tongue is heavily coated a slimy white colour. There is always a gastric connection with this remedy; the patient retches and vomits easily but is no better for vomiting, and there may be diarrhoea or constipation. They are worse for dry radiated heat.

Apis

The rash is slow to come out with this remedy. The face is very red and hot and the sufferer is worse for hot drinks and in a hot room. The eyelids are swollen and the face generally puffy. There is often delirium and/or shrieking out during sleep. Confluent eruptions can turn into oedematous swellings anywhere.

If there is delirium and/or calling out during sleep start with Apis 30, plussing it if necessary. Otherwise start with Apis 6.

Arsen. Album

This remedy is for restlessness and weakness with great sinking of strength. The eruption may have receded before coming out properly. There is an aggravation of the symptoms around midnight or soon after and sometimes this aggravation can happen around midday as well. They are thirsty but only have a few sips at a time, usually of something warm. They are icy cold and want to be kept well wrapped up although they always want fresh air as well. There can be vomiting and diarrhoea at the same time. Any pains are burning and better for warmth. They look sallow and there may be crusty eruptions around the mouth. They are frightened and do not like being alone.

Start with a 6, plussing it if necessary. You may well need to go up to Arsen. Album 30.

Belladonna

Here the face is red, dry and burning like Aconite, but the pupils are dilated; there is much less anxiety than with Aconite, but more grizzling, grumpiness, anger or irritability. Pains are throbbing but there still is the restlessness and thirst as with Aconite. They are worse at around 3 am or 3 pm and they keep themselves covered up as they are worse from a draught (whereas Aconite tosses off the covers). Although they seem hot and dry they are wet and sweaty under their clothes and hair. They are oversensitive, worse for noise and their eyes are worse for light so they want the curtains drawn. If the fever goes high they may well become delirious and/or twitchy.

Start by using Belladonna 6 but go up to a 30 if necessary and if there is real anger, irritability or twitchiness; you may need to plus the 30 or go up to a 200 if there is actual delirium.

Bryonia

The onset for this remedy is fairly slow. There is a dry, harsh cough and the face looks heavy and congested. Bryonia types are grumpy and want to be left alone and undisturbed, are better for lying still and worse for any motion. They desire cool air and are worse in a stuffy room; they tend to throw off the bedclothes. There is great thirst, dry mouth, tongue and lips. The rash is slow to come out or may start to recede before it has come out properly.

Start with Bryonia 6, plussing it if necessary, unless the fever is high and there is delirium, in which case use Bryonia 30 and possibly go up to a 200.

Euphrasia

Use this remedy if the eyes are the main or only problem; profuse hot burning tears from the eyes, photophobia, itching, redness, puffiness and a rash around the eyes. The nasal discharge is bland and may be profuse.

Give Euphrasia 6 at first and plus it if necessary. Occasionally a 30 may be required.

Gelsemium

This remedy is used particularly when measles comes on in warm summer weather or during a very mild winter. The onset is slow with shuddering chills up and down the spine. The limbs feel heavy, eyelids droop half closed; the sufferer feels weary and does not want to move. (This is different from Bryonia which does not want to move because of the pain.) There is no thirst.

Start with Gelsemium 6, plussing it if necessary. Often this is the only potency required.

Ipecac.

Ipecac. is used when there is constant nausea which is no better for vomiting. Also there is no thirst, a very clean tongue as well as exhaustion. The rash is slow coming out and usually there will be a dry cough, possibly wheezing with patients having difficulty getting their breath.

Kali Bich.

There can be violent stitching pains from the ear, or round about the ear which may extend to the roof of the mouth; as well as this there can be swelling of the ear, all around the ear and of the neck glands. There is a lot of discharge from the ear which can be smelly and is stringy or ropy. There may be deafness from catarrh blocking the eustachian tubes. There is a rattly cough with stringy expectoration and the voice may be hoarse. This remedy is usually needed later on in the disease.

Pulsatilla

With this remedy the patient wants lots of fuss and attention and does not want you to leave them. This is the opposite to Bryonia. Pulsatilla types are thirstless, weepy and clingy. There will be a lot of catarrh and a cough, which is loose during the day and may be dry at night. The lips are dry but there is no thirst. There may well be a dull earache, blocked eustachian tubes, and the eyes will itch and run.

Phosphorus

There is a violent, dry, exhausting cough; this cough and any hoarseness are worse talking, worse for cold, worse lying on the left side and there is a sense of a weight on the chest. There is nausea and they may vomit. They are very thirsty for cold water, have a high temperature and flushed cheeks. They are generally worse at twilight, worse in the dark, worse alone and extremely restless.

Sulphur

The two main symptoms for this remedy are that the rash is very itchy and they tend to be worse around 11am to about noon. It is useful when the rash is slow to come out and also for any symptoms which are slow to clear up once the disease is over. The other symptoms are the usual measles ones.

A BRIEF SUMMARY OF THE MAIN INDICATIONS FOR MEASLES REMEDIES

Catarrh:	Pulsatilla, Kali Bich.
Cough:	Pulsatilla, Kali Bich., Phos., Aconite, Bryonia
Cross/angry/irritable:	Antim. Crud., Bryonia, Bell.
Delirium:	Bell., Apis, Bryonia
Dry lips/mouth:	Bryonia, Pulsatilla
Early stages:	Aconite, Bell.
Ears affected:	Pulsatilla, Kali Bich.
Eyes affected particularly:	Euphrasia, Apis, Bell., Pulsatilla
Face, scabs/cracks round mouth, and nostrils:	Arsen. Album, Antim. Crud.

Fast onset:	Aconite, Bell.
Fearful/anxious:	Aconite, Arsen. Album
Itching:	Sulphur, Pulsatilla (eyes), Euphrasia (eyes)
Late stage:	Kali Bich., Sulphur
Pains in limbs:	Bryonia, Gels.
Receding rash or rash slow to come out:	Apis, Bryonia, Ipecac., Sulphur, Arsen. Album
Restlessness:	Arsen. Album, Bell., Phos.
Scabs/cracks round mouth/nostrils:	Arsen. Album, Antim. Crud.
Slow onset:	Bryonia, Gels.
Thirstless:	Antim. Crud., Ipecac.,Gels., Apis, Pulsatilla
Thirsty:	Bryonia (glass full), Aconite, Bell., Arsen. Album (sips), Phos.
Vomiting:	Antim. Crud., Ipecac., Phos., Aconite
Warm weather, summer, warm winters:	Gels.
Weepy, clingy:	Pulsatilla

Note: Never give more than one remedy at a time but be prepared to change the remedy if the symptoms change, although quite often only one remedy will be required. If you give a remedy because the rash is slow to come out or is receding before coming out properly, the rash should develop properly within a few hours. Unless I have stated otherwise, always start with a 6, going up in potency if necessary. Remember to stop the remedy as soon as there is improvement and restart only if the symptoms return.

PREVENTION

Like the other childhood diseases there are a variety of ways you can approach this and one of the following should suit:-

a) You could give Morbillinum 30, one dose once a year while your child is very young from the date your child would normally be given the MMR injection. Thereafter it is much better to let your child catch the illness and to treat it as described above or follow the advice in b) below.

b) You could give nothing at all unless there was a local outbreak of measles and then give Morbillinum 30 twice on one day initially then once every fourth day for three more doses; thereafter give one dose at fortnightly intervals until the danger is over. Alternatively Pulsatilla 6, morning and evening during an epidemic, can prevent many cases.

c) You could do both a) and b) above.

Personally I would not bother to do any prevention unless your child is very young or for a person who is not very strong in which case I would do b) above. Otherwise I would simply treat the patient once the illness was caught. That way the patient should obtain lifelong immunity, and with homoeopathic treatment the illness itself should be very mild.

41. Rubella or German Measles

One main worry about the rubella vaccine (part of the MMR vaccine) is that it appears to last such a short time. At the time of writing there have been quite a few cases of rubella locally and every child I have seen has had the vaccination; some of these children are only four years old. Thus women who think they are protected may prove not to be, and consequently run a very high risk of birth defects when pregnant if they come in contact with rubella. How much better it would have been if they had caught the disease naturally as children, so as to get genuine lifelong immunity. Also it is a medically accepted fact that one of the more immediate risks of the rubella vaccine is that it can cause arthritis in as many as 3 per cent of children (other statistics suggest this figure is in fact as high as 26 per cent of those vaccinated) and in over 12 per cent of adults. Again this vaccination is thought to increase the risk of auto-immune disease later in life (see section 36).

This disease can be so mild that people may not even know they have got it. The incubation period is from fourteen to twenty-one days. Early symptoms are similar to a mild flu type cold; headache, stiff muscles and runny nose. After two to three days there will be a faint pink rash which is almost flat, although some people develop a much brighter red rash. The rash is mostly on the trunk and can last anything from a few hours to a few days and may be accompanied by red, watery eyes and swollen glands at the back of the neck just below the hairline. **This is a very dangerous illness to get during the first few months of pregnancy as it can seriously damage the foetus. You should be extremely careful that you and your children when infectious avoid contact with anyone who may be pregnant.** (However, these days women usually have a blood test before getting pregnant so as to be able to have the vaccine again if they do not already have immunity.)

Aconite

Use this remedy if the patient is thirsty, restless, anxious or fearful. It is most indicated in the early stages of fever. Start with a 6 unless the restlessness and anxiety are extreme, in which case start with a 30.

Pulsatilla

Use this remedy when there is little or no thirst with the fever and a desire for open air; there is weepiness, dislike of being left alone and sadness.

Coffea

This remedy is indicated if there is extreme sleeplessness and sensitivity to noise, acuteness of all senses and excitability. You may want to start with a 12 or 30 if the symptoms are mostly Mentals.

PREVENTION

There are a variety of ways to prevent this disease and one of the following should suit your needs.

a) You could give Rubella 30, one dose annually from the time your baby would normally first have the MMR injection.

b) You could give Rubella 30 morning and evening on one day initially then one dose every fourth day for three more doses as soon as you heard of an outbreak locally; thereafter give one dose every two weeks until the danger is over.

c) You could give Pulsatilla 6 morning and evening for two weeks if there had been contact and/or if you heard of an outbreak locally.

d) You could do any combination of the above methods.

Although you have to be **very careful** about avoiding the risk of spreading the infection to someone who may be pregnant (please see above), it is preferable to let children catch this disease as they then have genuine lifelong protection and therefore run no risks during pregnancy themselves. It is much better to treat such a mild complaint once your child has actually got it.

SAFETY PRECAUTIONS FOR PREGNANCY

If you intend to have a baby and are not sure if you have had rubella it is very important to go to your doctor and be tested to see whether or not you have immunity. If you have not, your choice is either to have the rubella vaccine or else use homoeopathy; there are a variety of ways you can do this but the simplest is as follows: (1) you could take Rubella 30 one dose every fourth day for four doses *before* conception (you should repeat this at least every nine months if still not pregnant) and (2) then from conception onwards, until about the end of the fourth month, take Pulsatilla 30, one dose a fortnight (or else take Pulsatilla 6 twice a day for two weeks if there was rubella in the area and/or you were afraid you might have been in contact). It is wisest however, to deal with this prevention under the supervision of your homoeopath.

42. Diphtheria

This disease starts slowly with a headache and raised temperature and is characterized by a false membrane on any mucus surface, usually the throat, but sometimes inside the nose and occasionally on the skin. This membrane, most frequently covering the tonsils, is shiny, yellow-white-grey, and jelly-like. The breath is very smelly, the head aches, the throat is sore and the neck glands are swollen and painful. It is very infectious and can even be caught indirectly through sharing towels, drinking glasses or cutlery. Incubation period is from two to five days and it is rare to get this disease under one year of age. Cases of diphtheria had declined a great deal before the introduction of the diphtheria vaccine and it is a very rare disease now. Today it is mostly seen in the Third World.

Ailanthus Glandulosa

The tonsils have many deep angry looking ulcers and the throat is dark and swollen; the breath is very smelly. The tongue is dry and brown, the throat rough and scrapy, worse swallowing (possibly better for hot drinks rather than cold) and with a choking feeling; there is a dry hacking cough, drowsiness and maybe semi-consciousness.

Use a 30 from the beginning and plus it if necessary.

Apis

There is a great deal of oedema and inflammation with this remedy. The uvula (the small soft structure which hangs from the roof of the mouth above the root of the tongue) can look like a bag full of water with a lot of redness and puffiness. Any pains are stinging, worse swallowing, worse for hot food and drink and better for cool; generally there is very little thirst. There are dirty-greyish patches of membrane with the tonsils covered with deep grey ulcers, worse on the right side. Pains can extend to the ears and the breath is probably smelly. There can be oedematous swelling of the membrane lining the air passages and a sense of suffocation with high fever. Urination may be painful and scanty and the first sign that the remedy has begun to work will be an increased flow of urine.

Start with a 30 and go up if necessary.

Arsen. Album

Like Apis the Arsen. Album throat is oedematous but Arsen. Album has great thirst for warm or hot drinks, of which they only take sips each time. Just to be confusing the Arsen. Album throat can also look dry and shrivelled. Generally they feel very cold, want to be warm and well wrapped up, although they feel better for fresh air. Ulcers may well be on the roof of the mouth as well as in the throat; the tongue may be white and there may be a sensation of a hair in the throat. Blood may ooze from under the membrane. There may be urinary frequency, or scanty urine with burning pains, watery diarrhoea or constipation. They hate being alone and are incredibly restless as well as exhausted. They are often worse soon after midnight. This remedy is mostly indicated in later stages of the illness.

Start with a 6 and plus it but you may well need to go up to a 30.

Arum Triphyllum

This remedy is used in nasal diphtheria with a burning discharge from the nose; the mouth is full of red raised ulcers, is raw, red, sore and has a foul smell. The lips, nose and mouth are sore and bleeding. The throat is very raw and burning, worse swallowing, yet the sufferer wants to scratch it; they also want to pick at their nose even though it is so sore. Mentally they are cross and restless.

Start with a 6 and go up to a 30 if necessary.

Kali Bich.

This is another remedy to consider for nasal diphtheria. All discharges are ropy or stringy, tough and yellow or green. They hawk up thick mucus, the tonsils are swollen and the throat pains are worse on putting out the tongue and can extend to the neck and shoulders.

Lachesis

The membrane, soreness and pain start on the left and may spread to the right. The throat is a purple-red colour and is worse swallowing, worse for hot drinks and better for cold drinks. There is extreme sensitivity and they hate any pressure on their neck and throat, not wanting any clothing round it. There can be a kind of croupy cough which will wake them from sleep. The tongue often darts out in an attempt to lick the lips. There may be excessive cold, clammy perspiration. They tend to be chatterboxes even though their throat is so painful and they are frequently untrusting and suspicious.

Lac Caninum

The membrane and pain constantly change from side to side; the membrane can also start in the larynx and spread upwards into the mouth. The membrane is whitish and shiny and the tongue is coated with red edges. Saliva is dribbled and there may be cracks at the corners of the mouth. They are worse for empty swallowing and pains shoot to the ears. The pains are mostly sticking type pains; when swallowing, fluids can return through the nose. The skin is hyper-sensitive and worse for touch; they cannot bear even to let their fingers touch each other.

Lycopodium

Here the right side of the throat is affected first and it may move to the left side, the opposite direction to Lachesis. They are also better for warm drinks and worse for cold drinks which again is opposite to Lachesis. They wake cross and angry from sleep and they are generally worse from about 4 pm to about 8 pm. The tongue is dry, swollen, cracked and sufferers have to breathe through their mouth. The abdomen may be distended, uncomfortable and flatulent; urine may be decreased and/or with a red sandy sediment.

Merc. Cyanatus

This remedy has extreme weakness and prostration from the beginning, with blue face and cold extremities. They are extremely cold, tremulous and hardly able to stand. There is ulceration and the membrane is thick and grey-green, sometimes yellow; there are cutting pains in the throat, the breath is very offensive and there is profuse salivation. There can be profuse bleeding from the nose. There is also sweating without relief. It is best to start this remedy in a 30.

Phytolacca

There is a sensation of a hot ball or lump in the throat, which is very sore and painful on swallowing. The throat is dark reddish-blue and puffy and may have white-grey spots. The tongue has a fiery red tip but is heavily coated elsewhere and most of the pain is at the base of the tongue, particularly on putting it out. They are generally worse swallowing hot things. There may be aching of the head, back and limbs, with nausea, vertigo and faintness, particularly on sitting or standing up. Pains may extend to the ears when swallowing and there may also be smelly breath.

Diphtherinum

The patient seems extremely weak and tired from the very beginning and the usual more indicated remedies do not seem to be helping. The dark red swollen tonsils are painless and swallowing is not painful either. Nosebleeds, exhaustion, stupor, smelly breath and swollen glands are indicative symptoms. Use Diphtherinum 30.

PREVENTION

There are a number of ways to do this and one of the following should suit you:
a) Give Diphtherinum 30, one dose annually starting from the time your child would otherwise have been given the DPT inoculation.

b) Once you hear of an epidemic locally give Diphtherinum 30, morning and evening, on one day initially then one dose every fourth day for three more doses; thereafter one dose a fortnight. Continue for about six weeks or until the outbreak is over. You should also do this if you travel to a country where there is a risk of Diphtheria.

c) Do both a) and b) above.

I would only consider a) above for the very young but for anyone else I would just do b) above.

A BRIEF SUMMARY OF THE MAIN INDICATIONS FOR DIPHTHERIA REMEDIES

If you find this section on diphtheria and the number of remedies rather daunting remember that by giving the preventative Diphtherinum 30 described above you should usually prevent the onset of this disease; or if anyone does succumb to it they will most probably get it very mildly and it should seem as though they simply have a particularly nasty sore throat. I do not think you will find it hard to choose the homoeopathic remedy if you need to, but if necessary you should seek professional homoeopathic advice. Below is a brief summary of key symptoms and their remedies:

Abdomen distended:	Lycopodium
Back and limbs ache:	Phytolacca
Bleeding from lips/mouth:	Arum Triph., Arsen. Album
Bleeding from nose:	Merc. Cyanatus, Diphtherinum, Arum Triph.
Burning throat:	Arum Triph.
Chatterboxes:	Lachesis
Cold, extreme:	Merc. Cyanatus, Arsen. Album
Cool relieves:	Apis, Lachesis
Coma, semi-conscious:	Ailanthus Gland., Diphtherinum

Cough:	Ailanthus Gland., Lachesis
Cracks at mouth corners:	Lac Can.
Cracks on tongue:	Lycopodium
Discolouration of throat/membrane:	
dark:	Ailanthus Gland., Phytolacca
dirty greyish:	Apis
grey:	Phytolacca (spots), Merc. Cyanatus (and spots)
grey-green:	Merc. Cyanatus
purply red:	Lachesis, Apis
redness:	Apis, Arum Triph.
whitish:	Lac Can., Phytolacca (spots)
yellow:	Merc. Cyanatus
Dribbles:	Lac Can., Merc. Cyanatus
Drowsiness:	Ailanthus Gland., Diphtherinum
Dryness:	Lycopodium (tongue)
Ears, pains extending to:	Apis, Lac Can., Phytolacca
Face, blue:	Merc. Cyanatus
Face, cracks (mouth):	Lac Can.
Face, sore:	Arum Triph. (lips, nose, mouth)
Faintness/vertigo:	Phytolacca
Headache and backache:	Phytolacca
Hot lump sensation:	Phytolacca
Itching throat:	Arum Triph.
Later stages:	Arsen. Album
Left side worse:	Lachesis
Lick their lips:	Lachesis
Lump sensation, ball:	Phytolacca
Midnight, worse at:	Arsen. Album
Nasal diphtheria:	Arum Triph., Kali Bich.

Oedematous swelling:	Apis, Arsen. Album
and puffy:	Phytolacca
Pain, base of tongue:	Phytolacca (worse putting it out)
hot lump/ball:	Phytolacca
raw/burning:	Arum Triph.
rough/scrapy:	Ailanthus Gland.
shoots to ears:	Lac Can., Phytolacca
stinging:	Apis
worse putting tongue out:	Phytolacca, Kali Bich.
Painlessness of throat:	Diphtherinum
Pressure aggravates:	Lachesis
Restlessness:	Arum Triph., Arsen. Album
Right side worse:	Lycopodium
Ropy discharges:	Kali Bich.
Saliva profuse:	Merc. Cyanatus, Lac Can.
Scratches throat with tongue:	Arum Triph.
Side to side, changes:	Lac Can.
Skin hypersensitive:	Lac Can.
Smelly breath:	Ailanthus Gland., Arum Triph., Phytolacca, Merc. Cyanatus, Diptherinum
Soreness:	Arum Triph.
Sticking pains:	Lac Can.
Stinging pains:	Apis
Stringy discharges:	Kali Bich.
Suspicious:	Lachesis
Swallowing aggravates:	Ailanthus Gland., Arum Triph., Phytolacca, Apis, Lac Can., Lachesis
Sweating without relief:	Merc. Cyanatus

Swelling:

    generally: Apis, Arsen. Album, Diphtherinum

    abdomen: Lycopodium

    neck glands: Diphtherinum

    tongue: Lycopodium

    tonsils: Ailanthus Gland.

Thirst for cold drinks: Lachesis

Thirst for hot or warm drinks: Arsen. Album, Ailanthus Gland., Lycopodium

Thirstless: Apis

Time, worse from 4–8 pm: Lycopodium

    worse at midnight: Arsen. Album

Tongue:

    brown: Ailanthus Gland.

    coated base: Phytolacca (heavily)

    dry: Ailanthus Gland.

    hot: Ailanthus Gland.

    pain at base: Phytolacca

    puts it out: Lachesis

    red tip: Phytolacca

    white with red edge: Lac Can.

Ulcers: Ailanthus Gland. (deep), Arum Triph. (red), Phytolacca, Merc. Cyanatus, Diphtherinum

Urination painful: Apis

Urination increased: Lycopodium

Urine scanty: Apis, Lycopodium

Urine, sediment: Lycopodium

Warm drinks relieve: Ailanthus Gland., Arsen. Album (sips), Lycopodium

Warm/hot drinks aggravate: Lachesis, Phytolacca, Apis

Warmth relieves:	Lycopodium, Arsen. Album
Weakness, extreme:	Merc. Cyanatus, Diphtherinum, Arsen. Album

43. Whooping Cough

Statistics show that the pertussin vaccine (part of the DPT vaccine) does not work particularly well in preventing this disease and that there had been an 80 per cent decline in serious complications from whooping cough *prior* to the vaccine being introduced. Outbreaks of whooping cough have occurred when more than half of the sufferers have been vaccinated. The only age group seriously at risk when contracting whooping cough are the very young, or those already not very strong; they can usually be safely protected by using homoeopathy for prevention and/or treatment as described below. Known side effects (of the more immediate kind) from the DPT vaccine include anaphylactic shock (a life-threatening allergic reaction), continuous high-pitched screaming or wailing, and encephalitis. Other serious side effects which have not been ruled out include SIDS (cot deaths), juvenile diabetes, neurological damage, some forms of limb paralysis and poor concentration. Like the other vaccinations against childhood diseases there is evidence to show that the pertussin vaccine weakens the immune system and is a major contributing factor in the increase in auto-immune diseases (see section 36).

The incubation period for whooping cough is about seven days and the first or catarrhal stage looks very much like an ordinary slightly feverish cold and lasts about five days. The second or paroxysmal stage is then reached which is characterized by the paroxysms of coughing, with the mucus very hard to cough up. These spasms of coughing can go on and on until the sufferer may go rather blue and looks and sounds as if suffocating. The coughing spasm ends with a whoop, as they suck air into their lungs. The child often vomits at the end of a paroxysm. Untreated this phase can last over four weeks and then a less severe cough may follow for weeks or months. There may be nosebleeds or bloodshot eyes from the severity of the paroxysms of coughing. They are infectious for about three weeks after the onset of the spasmodic cough. Convulsions can be a complication and can last for half an hour or longer. These occur in about one case in half a million of (untreated) whooping cough cases. All these potentially serious symptoms should be avoidable with good care as well as good hygiene, diet and living standards; if homoeopathic treatment is used as well then the disease should not become serious and only last a short time. If necessary you should seek professional homoeopathic advice.

Pertussin 30

Take twice a day, stopping as soon as there is improvement, starting again if there is a slight relapse. This is the first and simplest remedy to think of. You should usually find you only need the remedy for a few days.

Drosera

This is a cough remedy which is particularly useful for whooping cough. It has the typical whooping cough type of cough with a time aggravation from midnight until three or four in the morning, and they are worse lying down. There is tickling and dryness in the throat which causes the spasmodic cough; the cough can go on and on until they vomit. They are better in fresh open air and worse when talking, laughing or swallowing. The nose may bleed from the violence of the cough and there may be hoarseness.

Ipecac.

Again this cough remedy can have the typical whooping cough symptoms but the main indication is if there is bleeding from the nose or mouth during coughing. There is a lot of rattling in the chest from mucus and they might manage to cough just a tiny bit up. There is a lot of nausea, which is no better for vomiting and with Ipecac. the tongue is always clean. They are better for open air. It is indicated if there are convulsions along with the other Ipecac. symptoms.

Bryonia

This cough occurs on the slightest movement; the patients eat or drink something and this starts them off coughing which is followed by vomiting. The spasmodic cough shakes the whole body and they tend to hold the chest while coughing. They are also very thirsty, worse for heat, worse deep breathing, better in open cool air and better for pressure.

Cuprum Metallicum

This cough is much better for cold drinks. It can be very violent and there can be vomiting, cramps, spasms and a purple face. It can be worse at 3 am and they cannot bear anything near the mouth. They often complain of having a metallic taste in the mouth.

PREVENTION

There are a variety of methods:-

a) You could give Pertussin 30, one dose annually while your child is young (up to about four years old) starting from the time your child would otherwise have been given the first Pertussin inoculation. Thereafter it is much better to let your child catch this disease and to treat it as described above or else follow the advice in b) below.

b) You could just give Pertussin 30 when you hear of an outbreak of whooping cough in your area. Here again there are a variety of ways of prescribing but it is probably best to give the remedy twice on one day initially, then one dose every fourth day for three more doses; thereafter give one dose every fourteen days or so until the outbreak is over.

c) You could do both systems a) and b) above.

Personally I would not bother with any prevention except for the very young or those who are not very strong, and then I would do b) above. Otherwise it is best to wait and treat them when they actually get the disease. That way they will obtain lifelong immunity; also any suffering should be much reduced as the illness should be very short with homoeopathic treatment during the disease itself.

44. Polio

There have been two types of polio vaccine with different side effects. The danger, as far as the live Oral Polio Vaccine, or OPV, is concerned, is that of contacts contracting the disease from the vaccine virus itself; this can be excreted through the mouth and the faeces for some weeks after the vaccination. Apparently this virus seems to cause the most virulent form of paralytic polio in those inadvertently in contact with it. Additional side effects (of the more immediate kind) from OPV are very poor weight gain as well as other paralytic diseases. The other vaccine, IPV or Inactivated Polio Vaccine, which was contaminated by another virus suspected of causing cancer, was used extensively during the 1950s and 1960s. Side effects of the IPV include various neurological complications as well as meningitis and encephalitis. Both OVP and IVP are currently in use.

The early stages of polio can easily be mistaken for flu. The symptoms can be sore throat, cold, headache, diarrhoea, vomiting, fever and pains in the limbs. The fever can drop to normal for a few days before rising again a second time. The spine can be very tender to touch and it can be difficult, painful, or stiff to bend, and there can be tremors of the muscles. A useful diagnostic test is that the patient is unable to kiss the knees because the back and neck are so tender, painful and stiff. (This test is also useful with meningitis.) The danger of this disease is the paralysis which can come on suddenly during the first couple of days. Early signs of this are (a) tremors and/or stiffness of muscles, and (b) coughing, spluttering and regurgitating liquids; all of which can be due to paralysis of the particular muscles involved. Incubation is usually from seven to twelve days although it can be as long as from five to thirty-five days. If treating this disease, you should seek professional homoeopathic advice if necessary.

Recently in the press there have been reports that those who have had polio in the past are sometimes developing symptoms of the disease many years later. In such cases there is no reason why the following remedies should not help them, if prescribed according to the symptom picture. I certainly have had patients who have had polio many years ago and whenever they have a fever the symptoms have been very similar to when they originally had the disease; they have taken whichever of the following remedies was most indicated with great success.

Lathyrus Sativus 30

All paralysis from polio is supposed to be preventable by using this remedy. (Ref. Dr. Grimmer of Chicago in the 1930s and Dr. Dorothy Shepherd in 1967 in *Homoeopathy in Epidemic Diseases*.) Give Lathyrus Sativus 30 morning and evening on one day at fortnightly intervals from the moment you hear of any cases locally, and it should be very unlikely that the disease will be caught at all however close or frequent the contact. If the disease has been caught and there is already some tremor, tenderness and/or stiffness of the muscles, give Lathyrus Sativus 30 about every forty minutes, stopping as soon as improvement sets in. It is unlikely that you will need to give more than a few doses; patients will most probably fall asleep and be a great deal better when they wake up. Repeat the remedy if or whenever the symptoms return.

Gelsemium

With this remedy there is great anticipatory fear of the disease and its consequences, as well as trembling and lethargy. It can be used to treat the disease itself in the early stages and also to prevent its onset. The fever symptoms are accompanied by heaviness of the head, eyelids and limbs. There is shaking and shuddering during chill and heat; tremors, weakness and heaviness. The headache is better for profuse urination and there is no thirst even during the fever. There may be difficulty swallowing and food as well as drink may be regurgitated because of muscle weakness or paralysis. This remedy is particularly indicated in warm, mild, damp weather; the English summer or early autumn. Start with Gelsemium 12.

Eupatorium Perf.

This remedy is indicated when there is a severe bruised or aching pain of the limbs and back. It feels 'as if the bones were broken' and they dare not move for the pain. There is shivering and shaking during the chill. They are better for vomiting and worse for motion, worse for cold air, worse periodically and worse from 7–9 am. Like Gelsemium, Eupatorium Perf. is most indicated in the early stages of the disease preventing more serious developments. Start with a 12.

Physostigma

There is weakness and tremors of the muscles, particularly of the lower back and limbs, which do not respond to the will. Also there are contracted pupils and twitching of eye muscles. Generally they are worse for cold, worse for cold water even to the point of dreading it, and worse for draughts. Any paralysis and numbness is worse on the left side and the gait is ataxic - shaky and uncoordinated. Start with a 12.

Belladonna

The onset is fast and the patient is burning hot. The skin is red and dry but is probably damp and sweaty under the hair and under the clothes or bedclothes. The pupils are dilated and their eyes are worse for light. They are worse for draughts. They are usually angry and irritable, or at least grumpy and difficult. They are hypersensitive and are worse for any noise. They are worse, or the symptoms come on initially, at around 3 am or 3 pm. They are thirsty particularly for lemonade. If they can they prefer to be lying half propped against the pillows particularly if they have a headache. Pains are throbbing or pulsating, cramping or spasmodic. If the temperature goes really high there can be delirium with a great deal of restlessness. They have cold extremities, weak and tottering gait, jerks and spasms in the limbs with a heavy paralytic feeling. The back can feel broken, with stiffness of the neck and back. Start with Belladonna 6 or 12 unless the patient is very cross and/or restless in which case start with Belladonna 30; you may need to go up to a 200 particularly if there is delirium.

PREVENTION

a) You could give Polio 30, one dose annually starting at the time your baby would normally be given the first vaccine against polio, whether OPV or IPV.

b) If there is an outbreak locally or if travelling to areas where polio could be a problem, I would give Lathyrus Sativus 30 morning and evening on one day initially then one dose every fourth day for three more doses; thereafter one dose a fortnight until the scare is over.

Personally I would consider doing a) above for the very young and b) otherwise. If there has been possible contact with newly vaccinated babies, perhaps in a swimming bath, I would do a) and/or b) plus regular constitutional homoeopathic treatment.

45. Meningitis

The following details about this disease are given so that you will find it easier to recognize in order to get help urgently. While it is useful to know that this type of serious disease can be treated successfully with homoeopathy, it is important to realize that, due to its speed and severity there is no time to lose and for this reason it is very unwise to attempt to treat it yourself. *The most important thing is to seek professional help and not to waste any time.*

Meningitis is inflammation of the membranes of the spinal cord and/or brain. It begins with a fever, loss of appetite, constipation and headache. The eyes are worse for light and sufferers are intolerant of noise. It can lead to delirium, stiff neck and convulsions. In children the only obvious signs may be the raised temperature, vomiting and sometimes convulsions. A diagnostic test for meningitis is to see if the patient is able to 'kiss his knees' which he will be unable to do due to pain and stiffness in the neck. With the fever and headache there will most likely be vomiting and sometimes a pink, spotty rash may develop on the body. We are all frequently reminded about 'the glass test' for this rash, which should indicate whether or not it is meningitis. Simply press a glass against the skin over the rash area and if the spots do **not** disappear with pressure then that indicates meningitis. However, it is very important to realize that someone can have meningitis without having the rash, and that the rash often only occurs later on in the disease. Apart from the glass test demonstrating the rash, three important indicators that this disease may be present are:-

1) the *extreme* degree of pain from the headache, with a fever and usually with vomiting;
2) the *speed* with which the symptoms come on and with which the patient seems to deteriorate;
3) the *stiffness and pain* of the neck, and the patients are unable to kiss their knees.

Any of the above symptoms should alert you to the possibility of meningitis and to get help immediately.

There are now newer vaccines against meningitis and some degree of prevention is possible using the homoeopathic Meningitis Nosode and potentized vaccine described below. Meningitis can affect all age groups but babies are at high risk. Well nourished children from about 5 years old are not at particularly high risk but teenagers and young adults are again at high risk because it can be spread via saliva when kissing; this is probably why it occurs most frequently in those at secondary school and university.

PREVENTION

The best remedy to get is a *mixture* of the following:-
Meningococcus Nosode 30, with the latest Meningitis C Vaccine 30.

This can be obtained from Helios Homoeopathic Pharmacy (see page 211).

Possible prescribing methods for meningitis prevention are:-

a) Give the meningitis mixture as described above, one dose annually starting from the time the baby would otherwise have been given the meningitis inoculation.

b) If there are any cases of meningitis locally give the remedy morning and evening, on one day initially, then one dose every fourth day for three more doses; thereafter one dose a fortnight until the danger is over.

c) If you feel your child is going to be in a high risk situation or is at a high risk age, then give the remedy more frequently, perhaps 3-6 monthly depending on the situation and their behaviour.

d) Avoid as much as possible the situations which increase susceptibility to the disease, (see Susceptibility below). If someone is at risk due to one of these reasons and is also showing symptoms which could be meningitis, give the meningitis preventative mixture exactly as described in b) above. This should be done as well as any other indicated homoeopathic treatment for them.

e) If you are not vaccinating your children against this disease you should make sure that they have constitutional homoeopathic treatment reasonably regularly so that their health is as good as possible. Combining this with the meningitis prevention described above should increase anyone's resistance to the illness and decrease susceptibility to it.

As I have mentioned previously this disease can be very dangerous because of the speed with which the patient can deteriorate. There is no time to waste so obviously it is best not to attempt to treat it yourself. If you are in the lucky position of having *immediate* access to a professional homoeopath and have *all* the possible remedies indicated in a wide range of potencies at hand, then it may just be worth considering. If you cannot get *immediate homoeopathic help* you should always have allopathic treatment *at once*. The following remedy details for this illness are given to inform the layperson that this type of serious disease *can* be treated successfully with homoeopathy, not really on the understanding that he or she will actually try it without professional homoeopathic assistance.

SUSCEPTIBILITY

From a *holistic* point of view all the following conditions and situations can increase someone's *susceptibility* to meningitis and should be avoidable with a mixture of common sense and homoeopathic treatment. These can be sunstroke, suppression of a skin rash, (for example during the acute childhood diseases as well as in chronic diseases) or suppression of any inflammatory rash, suppression of a fever, suppression of any discharge or sweat, suppression of an ear discharge, suppression of a nasal discharge, and after a head injury, spinal injury or other wound. If you are not vaccinating your children it is very important to realize that you must give them homoeopathic treatment whenever they get the childhood diseases so as to avoid any complications, one of which could be meningitis. You should also bear in mind that meningitis is known to be one of the many side effects from other vaccinations, particularly DPT and MMR, so that if you do not immunize your children against those other diseases the subsequent risk of meningitis is reduced.

If homoeopathic remedies are used to cure sunstroke, the cure goes with, rather than against the curative action of the body, so meningitis is less likely to occur. If homoeopathic remedies are used to treat all the acute childhood diseases then there will be no suppression of discharges or of rashes and there should be much less risk of meningitis occurring. If any fever, or localized inflammation is cured by homoeopathic remedies, rather than suppressed with ordinary medicine, again there is much less likely to be a risk of meningitis, due to the homoeopathic treatment going along with the natural direction of cure of the body. If homoeopathic remedies are given during the treatment of head injuries, spinal injuries, and other wounds, rather than ordinary painkillers etc., then amongst other things pain, shock and any internal bleeding should be stopped as well as the susceptibility to meningitis being reduced. In all the above situations the homoeopathic treatment and advice given in this book under the different sections should greatly reduce the risk of getting the disease in the first place. In other words susceptibility is reduced and the complications, which can lead to meningitis, are much less likely to occur if homoeopathic remedies are used for these conditions. The incidence of this disease has increased a great deal in recent years; this may well be attributable to the fact that children's vitality has been weakened more than ever by having had so many childhood inoculations, and other suppressive treatments.

I have included symptom pictures for a few remedies which are most commonly indicated for meningitis and with which you are likely to be familiar, as they are used elsewhere in this book for other ailments. There are numerous other remedies which a professional homoeopath would consider alongside these. With the intensity and energy of the fever along with the delirium, the potencies required will probably be high, such as a 200 or 10M, not the middle to low range of potencies described in this book and which you may have at home. Remedies may need to be repeated more frequently as any high fevers might burn up the remedy quickly.

Aconite

The onset of meningitis needing Aconite can be triggered by checked perspiration, internal injury, anger, fright, strong emotions, or too much sun; particularly from falling asleep in the sun. The onset is usually very sudden; sufferers are better for uncovering and coolness, worse around 9 pm or 9 am, very thirsty, their eyes will be worse for light and the pupils usually contracted. There can be numbness, powerlessness and coldness of the limbs, hands and feet; also cutting pains in the lower limbs. There can be tingling, pricking or crawling sensations in the back but particularly in the spine. The face looks anxious and is mostly very red, hot and dry although it can go very pale on sitting up; occasionally the face can be bright red on one side and pale on the other. Head pains are worse in the forehead and are violent, bursting, and burning in particular. Mentally they are extremely fearful, anxious and restless and think they will die. The fever is usually very high and the patient is burning hot, dry and red, often with delirium.

If there is delirium start with Aconite 200, otherwise start with Aconite 30. Remember that with a very high fever the remedy needs more frequent repetition, but always prescribe according to the advice in section 10; improvement follows very quickly after giving the remedy.

Apis

This is a remedy which often follows Belladonna well in meningitis. It is more often indicated for young babies than for older children and adults. It often follows the suppression or slow spread of an inflammatory skin eruption, which may occur during some infectious disease, or perhaps suppression by vaccination. The patients may bore their head into the pillow (like Belladonna) and roll the head from side to side. The face and head are congested and the sufferer shrieks out during sleep or is unconscious but making single, sharp screams. Urine may be scanty but with frequent desire to pass it; there is no thirst despite a very dry mouth with a possibly dry blistered tongue, but occasionally they may want and be better for milk. They are worse for touch, motion and heat in any way. Mentally they may be extremely restless or they appear to be in a complete stupor and may not respond even to light or noise. There may be oedema anywhere on the skin as well as very red spots like nettlerash.

Start with Apis 30 but you may need to go up to a 200 quite soon.

Arnica

This meningitis may well follow a trauma or injury of some kind, although it may not occur until some days or weeks following the trauma. The face and head are hot and red while the rest of the body is very cold. They cringe and move away if anyone touches them even if they are unconscious. They may scream out while unconscious and bore the head into the pillow. The neck muscles are very weak and can scarcely support the head; the neck is also worse for any touch or pressure. There can be nervous twitching even during heavy sleep.

There may be involuntary defecation or micturition.

It is always best to start with Arnica 30 here. You may need to go up to a 200 or higher.

Belladonna

This is one of the most frequently indicated remedies for meningitis. Again like Aconite the onset is sudden. Susceptibility is increased following exposure to cold, wet, windy weather, very hot sun or during dentition. The sufferer is very sensitive to noise, draughts and light, the pupils are dilated and the conjunctivae are very red. The face may have an angry, furious look, be bright red and very hot; the veins of the face and head are swollen and throbbing, and while the head is very hot the rest of the body and extremities may be very cold. While they are generally very dry there can be sweating under the clothes and hair. The headache is stupefying and pulsating, spreading from the neck up into the head and is better when bending the head backwards; the patient bores his head into the pillow although the headache itself is much worse for movement. Mentally they are at best grumpy but usually angry, irritable or fairly cross. Convulsions can shake the whole body, distort the face and are worse from the slightest touch or from light. There can be throbbing and burning pains in the spine as well as shocks, spasms and twitching in the arms and legs. With delirium there can be biting, muttering and moaning, as well as the patient seeing horrid visions, monsters or faces.

Start with Belladonna 30 or 200 but if there is delirium a 200 or higher will be needed. There should be improvement within minutes of giving the remedy.

Bryonia

This meningitis may come on from the suppression of a rash or eruption of some kind. It is another remedy which often follows Belladonna well in meningitis. The patient appears to be constantly moving the jaws as though he were chewing something. Dryness runs through many of the symptoms; the mouth is parched and dry with painful dry sore lips and great thirst; stools are dry or he is constipated; urination may be suppressed or painful. Any pains are stitching and are worse for the slightest motion. The joints and neck may be stiff and the headache is splitting. The eyes may be squinting and the face dark red and bloated looking. Their mood can alternate between being hasty, rash and impetuous, with being delirious, sluggish and stuporous. They are nauseous and feel faint on the slightest motion.

Start with Bryonia 30 unless there is delirium when you may need to start with a 200.

Gelsemium

This meningitis can occur during dentition or from exposure to the sun. There is extraordinary weakness and exhaustion; the patients can only stagger rather than walk and are very uncoordinated, vision is blurred, they cannot hold the head up properly, nor can they speak clearly. The eyelids droop half open and the hands and feet are icy cold while the rest of the body is hot and congested. There is no thirst and there is nausea, giddiness and vomiting. These symptoms are more likely to occur during mild warm weather.

Start with Gelsemium 6 or 12, and you may have to go up to a 30. The energy with this remedy is so low and the patient so weak that you may not need to go up to a 200.

Glonoine

The head feels enlarged, in fact it feels enormous; there are throbbing pains and the head is worse for movement. The eyes are red, the patient sees black spots before the eyes; the pulse is fast and shakes the whole body or at the very least is felt strongly in the head and chest; pain tends to ascend to the head from the chest and neck. There is nausea, spasmodic vomiting, trembling and twitching, convulsions and heavy sleep from which it is difficult to wake them. They are relieved by cool things, worse bending the head back, better sitting still but want to be propped up because lying down makes them feel much worse. They are worse for motion and sit holding the head still, but do not want any other pressure on their head. Meningitis needing Glonoine can be caused by sunstroke.

Rhus Tox.

This remedy is indicated when meningitis occurs following the suppression or non-appearance of an eruption during some other infectious disease, as well as from getting wet or sleeping on damp ground, which can happen when people go camping. It can also be caused when people are hot and sweaty from playing a strenuous game and instead of getting dry and changed, hang around in that damp state getting cold. There are tearing pains and stiffness in the muscles and joints, which are worse for damp and cold and better for lying or pressing against something hard. There is vertigo and staggering and the head feels like a weight which they can hardly hold up. The headache feels bruised and extends to the ears and can be accompanied by bleeding from the ears and/or nose. Mentally they are extremely anxious, restless and despairing, and are beside themselves with the pains.

Start with Rhus Tox. 30, and you may need to go up to a 200 or higher.

46. A final note on general prevention

If you wish to give homoeopathic preventative remedies annually for the acute childhood diseases while your children are still very young, which I have indicated as one of the choices in each section, you may find it easier to combine some of the remedies. By this I mean that instead of the DPT injection and polio oral vaccine you could give one dose of Diphtherinum 30 combined with Pertussin 30 and Polio 30 (and possibly Tetanus 30, although you should see section 15 for advice about preventing Tetanus, which I think is preferable to taking Tetanus 30 routinely); or instead of the MMR injection you could give Morbillinum 30 combined with Parotidinum 30 and Rubella 30.

It is probably better, however, to give the remedies separately, in which case a four week interval between each one is about right. However, most people just want to protect their children from the four most serious diseases. A good method is to give in rotation on the first day of each month Pertussin 30, then Polio 30, then Morbillinum 30 and then Meningitis 30; this should be followed by some months without any nosodes, then you should start doing the sequence again. It is important to have constitutional treatment as well, so as to increase the general level of health and resistance to disease. When children get a bit older many parents prefer their children to get whooping cough and measles in order to get genuine lifelong immunity from these diseases. The two diseases that people then remain most anxious about are polio and meningitis. There is no reason why you should not go on giving the homoeopathic prevention for these two fairly routinely; so follow the individual recommendations in this chapter suitable for the risk level for both diseases. It does not matter which method you choose but whatever you do **you must keep a written record for each member of your family in a safe place.** This is very important so that you know exactly what you have done and when you should give the next dose. You must also remember to avoid all the things which can antidote homoeopathic remedies when doing any long-term prevention, see section 8.

Apart from polio, smallpox and meningitis, remember that it is important actually to get these childhood diseases once children are old enough and fit enough; not only so as to obtain lifelong immunity, but also to throw off to some extent the miasmatic weaknesses which we all inherit. Perhaps the only time when it might be considered essential to give the homoeopathic preventatives would be when someone is already weakened with some other chronic illness or when a child is very young, depending on the particular disease. It is also **very important** to remember that your family should also have a good diet, not live off junk food, and get regular constitutional homoeopathic treatment. This means that they will be as fit and well as possible so that they will be able to cope with these diseases better when they catch them. If you yourself have not had some of these diseases, you must remember that you may no longer be immune despite having been vaccinated; so when your children actually get any of these diseases you should either protect yourself with homoeopathy, or be prepared to get and treat the disease concerned. You must also bear in mind that they tend to be more unpleasant to get as an adult, (but having homoeo-pathic treatment should help with this).

At the time of writing, these are what are known as 'notifiable diseases' so if any of your family get any of them, you *must* report this to your doctor. If your doctor actually sees the patient during one of these diseases when you have been using homoeopathy, you may well find that the doctor will find it difficult to agree a diagnosis. The reason for this is that, although there may be the physical symptoms of the disease present, the patient will not be suffering very much, which will seem very unusual indeed to a doctor if he is not accustomed to the benefits of homoeopathic remedies.

The homoeopathic remedies Diphtherinum 30, Pertussin 30, Morbillinum 30, Parotidinum 30, Rubella 30, Meningitis 30, Polio 30, Tetanus 30, Varicella 30 and Variolinum 30 are known as nosodes and are made out of the actual disease product concerned, and are best used for prevention. They are potentized up to the 30C potency; this means that there is no single molecule of the disease product left in the remedy so it is perfectly safe to take.

Chapter Five

HOMOEOPATHY
WHEN TRAVELLING

47. *Malaria*

Before working out which preventative treatment you should take for malaria it is important to find out whether you are going to a high or low risk area. Rainy seasons and marshy, swampy low-lying areas are traditionally the times and places for malaria to be most prevalent, so the level of risk depends very much upon the time of year and the altitude. There are many urban areas as well as high altitude areas which are often free from malaria and in these places there is less need to take prevention. It is well worth checking the risk factors on the internet for the area to which you are travelling. Over the years some anti-malarial drugs seem to have become less effective because some parasites have become drug resistant. Although the latest drug, Lariam, has been successful in dealing with malaria, it is reported to have many serious, unpleasant and lasting side effects; people have become anxious about the risk of taking it because the side effects can be so horrible.

HOMOEOPATHIC PREVENTION FOR BOTH TYPES OF MALARIA

No preventative methods are 100% reliable against malaria, whether allopathic or homoeopathic, but the following are good and well worth trying; they are not as complicated as they may at first seem. They are also preferable to the possibility of getting the side effects from allopathic drugs. You should choose whichever one of the following regimes suits you best according to the length of time you will be in a malarial area, and also according to your susceptibility to getting bitten generally.

For a short break of a few days, less than a week:

Malaria 30   should be taken one dose in the morning and evening on one day each week. Start the Malaria 30 two weeks before travelling to a suspect area and continue for three weeks afterwards.

Sea Salt 30   should be taken one dose in the morning and evening on the day you arrive only.

China 6   should be taken one dose in the morning and evening starting the second day you are away and continued daily while you are there.

Staphisagria 30   should be taken one dose in the late afternoon or early evening every day if you are the sort of person who gets bitten easily, or on alternate days if you are not. Start this the day before you arrive.

For a 1–2 week holiday:

Malaria 30   should be taken one dose in the morning and evening on one day each week, perhaps Sundays. Start the Malaria 30 two weeks before travelling to a suspect area and continue for three weeks after you arrive home.

Sea Salt 30   should be taken one dose in the morning and evening on one day midweek, perhaps Wednesdays.

China 6   should be taken one dose in the morning and evening on all the remaining days, that is every day except Sundays and Wednesdays (or whichever days you are taking the Malaria 30 and Sea Salt 30).

(You only need take the China 6 and the Sea Salt 30 while you are in the malarial areas. You do not have to start them beforehand like you do with the Malaria 30.)

Staphisagria 30   should be taken one dose in the early evening or late afternoon on alternate days starting the day before you get to a malarial area.

If you tend to get bitten very easily take the Staphisagria 30 daily for the first three to five days, and then take it every alternate day thereafter. If you are the type of person who seldom gets bitten, take it every third day.

For a 2–8 week holiday:

Malaria 30   should be taken one dose in the morning and evening on one day each week, perhaps Sundays. Start the Malaria 30 two weeks before travelling to a suspect area and continue for three weeks after you arrive home.

Sea Salt 30   should be taken one dose in the morning and evening on one day midweek, perhaps Wednesdays.

China 6   should be taken one dose in the morning and evening on all the remaining days, that is every day except Sundays and Wednesdays (or whichever days you take the Malaria 30 and Sea Salt 30).

(You only need take the China 6 and the Sea Salt 30 while you are in the malarial areas. You do not have to start them beforehand like you do with the Malaria 30.)

Staphisagria 30   should be taken one dose in the early evening or late afternoon on alternate days starting the day before you get to a malarial area. You do this for the first two weeks; after that take it twice a week for the third, fourth and fifth weeks, then once a week for the sixth, seventh and eighth weeks. If you think it is a very high risk area or season continue taking it twice a week throughout.

If you get bitten very easily indeed you could take it daily for the first three days, then take it every alternate day for the next two weeks and then you should take it twice a week for the remaining weeks.

For 8 weeks – 6 months:

Malaria 30   Do the first two months as described above. Then decrease the frequency of the Malaria 30 one in the morning and evening from once a week to once every two weeks for the third and fourth months, then once every three weeks for the remaining time. If the risk is very high continue taking it on one day every two weeks.

Sea Salt 30   Take Sea Salt 30, one in the morning and evening one day midweek, perhaps Wednesdays, for the first two months. Then take it once every two weeks for the third and fourth months decreasing to once every three weeks for the remaining time. If the risk is very high continue taking it on one day every two weeks.

China 6   should be taken one dose in the morning and evening on all the remaining days; that is every day except for the days you are taking Malaria 30 or Sea Salt 30. However, about every sixth week you should have a break off the China 6 completely for five consecutive days; it would be best to do this from Sunday to Thursday inclusive, starting again on the Friday, (that is if you are taking Malaria 30 on Sundays and Sea Salt 30 on Wednesdays).

Staphisagria 30 should be done as above for the first two months. Then decrease the frequency to once a week for the remaining time.

Longer than 6 months:

You should do the first six months as described above, then continue as if you were still in the fifth and sixth months. However, such a long length of time will usually mean that you will be there during a low risk season or might be travelling to lower risk places. *At such times it is important to give yourself a complete break off the remedies whenever you can.* If you only have a short break off the remedies of anything up to about two weeks, then when you return to a malarial area you should go back onto the regime you were on before you had the break. If on the other hand you managed to have a much longer time off the remedies you should start again at the beginning if the risk is high; if the risk is low you should start as if you were in week three of the 2-8 week regime, or the third month of the 8 week to 6 month regime depending on the risk factors.

GENERAL PREVENTION ADVICE

Apart from taking the preventative homoeopathic remedies it is very important that you use Pyrethrum Ø to stop the mosquitoes from biting you *instead of* any of the conventional medical smelly sprays. The conventional sprays, creams and burners *must not be used if they contain substances which antidote homoeopathic remedies.* If you used them it would spoil all your efforts in taking the homoeopathic remedies. Pyrethrum Ø does not affect the homoeopathic remedies and you can get this as a spray from homoeopathic pharmacies, or you could get the Ø in a 100ml bottle and dab it on your wrists, ankles and neck etc., which is a less expensive way of using it. Pyrethrum is not only supposed to stop you getting bitten in the first place but is cooling and prevents itching when dabbed onto bites, see section 18, 'Bites and stings'. There are also other sprays which homoeopathic pharmacies have which you could try, just make sure they do not contain anything which can antidote your homoeopathic remedies. It is very important to sleep inside a mosquito net soaked in Pyrethrum as well as keeping as much of the body covered up as possible, particularly in the evenings. Remember also to avoid all the medicaments and other things which can make the homoeopathic remedies inefficient, or even may antidote them, (see sections 6 and 8). It is helpful to consult your homoeopath before going to malarial areas because there are other remedies for dealing with the long-term susceptibility to getting bitten and consequently to malaria. If you had homoeopathic constitutional treatment it would increase your resistance and decrease your susceptibility to getting not only malaria but other diseases as well.

INTRODUCTION TO TREATING MALARIA

Malaria, particularly the more severe kind, cerebral malaria, which is caused by *Plasmodium falciparum*, can be very dangerous partly because of the speed with which the patient can sink. Both kinds are particularly dangerous for pregnant women and young children. As there is no time to waste it is obviously best not to attempt to treat it yourself. If you cannot get *immediate* homoeopathic help you should always have allopathic treatment and *not waste any time.* The following remedy details for this illness are given so as to inform the layperson that this type of serious disease can be treated successfully with homoeopathy, not on the understanding that he or she will actually try it without professional help.

The general symptoms may include rigor (shivering fit/chill), headache, intense fever delirium, sweating, diarrhoea, vomiting, cough, malaise, muscle pains, jaundice (yellow skin/yellow whites of eyes).

SYMPTOMS AND TREATMENT FOR THE LESS SEVERE TYPE OF MALARIA, ALSO KNOWN AS BENIGN MALARIA

When the female mosquito, which has been infected with the malaria parasite, bites someone, the parasites go to the liver where they multiply fast and then travel back into the bloodstream. The bouts of malaria occur whenever the parasites are released into the bloodstream, destroying the young and the old red blood cells. Usually in benign malaria the parasites multiply at intervals. Although this is the less severe and less virulent kind of malaria, it is nevertheless serious and exhausting. The incubation period varies between 8 to 14 days but can be delayed much longer depending on the type of parasite and also if conventional prophylactic drugs have been taken. Apart from the above general symptoms the sequence of events is usually as follows:-

Recurrent attacks lasting a few hours or days, start suddenly with a cold phase of violent shivers and shakes lasting up to one hour or a bit more. These are followed by a hot phase with a temperature as high as 41°C with thirst, abdominal pain, vomiting, increased urine, delirium, and flushed face and may last up to six hours. The sweating phase then begins lasting up to about two hours. These phases can recur every two to four days depending on the type of parasite and the whole cycle leaves the patient exhausted.

Eup. Perf.

Severe aching bone pains indicate the need for this remedy. The chilly phase often is worse around 7-9 am. There is nausea and vomiting as the cold/shivering phase passes. There is heaviness/pressure over the skull/forehead. The sweating phase is virtually absent.

Gelsemium

Gelsemium is needed for a flushed face during the hot phase. There is no thirst. The muscles feel bruised. Chills and shivers run up and down the back. There is a great deal of shaking, trembling and weakness.

Rhus Tox.

There is nettlerash/urticaria with itching and restlessness during the hot phase. This goes as the sweating phase starts. There are yellow watery stools in the hot phase. Any joint and muscle pains are worse for initial motion but better for continued motion. (Do not confuse this remedy with Eup. Perf. which has very severe bone pains but without this modality.)

Apis

The cold phase starts with sudden violent vomiting. Nettlerash/urticaria may spread over the head and body as the cold phase subsides.

Often there may be swelling of the lips and face. Any joint pains may be severe. The chill may be worse at 3 pm or 3 am and patients are always worse in a warm room and for any external heat. (This is opposite to Belladonna, although Belladonna is also worse around 3 pm or 3 am.)

China

There is ringing in the ears during the cold phase. The spine is tender, worse for touch and pressure. There is marked periodicity of the attacks, always coming precisely at a particular time of day or night, or else coming every two days or whatever it may be. There is never any thirst except possibly during the change over from the cold to hot stage. While many of the symptoms, particularly the sweats, may be worse at night, the fever seldom returns at night.

Ipecac.

This remedy is indicated for extreme constant nausea. The patient usually has a very clean red tongue which is unusual with such nausea. Only very occasionally it may have a thick coating of yellow. There is increased saliva. The chill stage is slight but the heat stage is extreme. There is nearly always a feeling of weight and pressure on the chest.

Arsen. Album

The patient is extremely restless, feeling as if driven to moving from place to place. There is neuralgia on one side of face or head, with maddening pain. They feel faint and sleepy before an attack. They feel better for external heat, are thirsty for little and often, preferring warm drinks. Pains are burning and better for warmth. The extreme weakness is out of proportion to the symptoms. One of the phases may be missed out. Diarrhoea and vomiting may occur at the same time, so that the patient does not know whether to sit on the lavatory or have his head over it.

Pulsatilla

This patient may be thirsty during the chilly phase, although normally they are thirstless despite the fact that the mouth feels dry. The symptoms and modalities may be very changeable. No two phases are alike. They are happy one minute but miserable the next. They need cool air even if the body is cold, although the head may be hot. Sweats may be one-sided only. There could be an aggravation towards the evening.

Nux Vomica

Here there is external chilliness with internal heat or vice versa. During the chill they are either very thirsty or quite thirstless, but in both cases they are not relieved by drinking. The abdomen is distended and uncomfortable with any gastric and bilious symptoms. They are cross, anguished, and delirious. They desire to be covered, even during the heat stage and sweat stage. They have burning of the hands, ears and face during the heat phase but blueness during the chilly phase.

REMEDIES FOR CONFUSED CASES

You should compare the above remedies with the more detailed descriptions elsewhere in this book, particularly in section 23 on 'Fevers' and in the Materia Medica in the final chapter, to help you choose. Normally with this kind of severe acute disease the symptom picture is clearly defined, making it easier to choose the homoeopathic remedy. However, if the symptoms are very unclear some homoeopaths suggest the following way of prescribing:

Alternate Nux Vom. 30, Arsen. Album 30 and Puls. 30, one dose every 30 minutes to about two hourly. Start with Nux Vom. if you start during a cold phase, otherwise you should start with Arsen. Album.

This way of prescribing will help up to a point; you will then find that the true remedy picture will emerge and you can then prescribe the remedy that is more clearly indicated, with *much* better and faster results.

For cases which are totally unresponsive and/or which have been confused by giving allopathic drugs as well, wait till an attack is over and then give one dose every hour of Natrum Mur. 200 for 3-6 doses. This again should result in making the case much clearer and you should then be able to choose the correct remedy during the next attack. If the symptom picture still remains unclear then repeat the Natrum Mur. after the next attack is over. The occasional intercurrent dose of Malaria 30 will always help.

SYMPTOMS AND TREATMENT FOR THE MORE SEVERE TYPE OF MALARIA CAUSED BY *PLASMODIUM FALCIPARUM*, ALSO KNOWN AS CEREBRAL MALARIA

This is mostly found in West Africa and is the kind which causes most deaths. The incubation period is 9-14 days, but can be as long as one month, or may be longer if prophylactic drugs have been taken. This more serious type could cause death within hours; the periodicity is not marked (though it can sometimes be every third day), as this type of malaria usually consists of one very serious bout of the disease. This is because after the parasites multiply in the liver they are then released back into the bloodstream all at once destroying all red blood cells (not just destroying young and old blood cells, as in benign malaria). Red blood cells become sticky and may block blood vessels in vital organs. The most common symptoms are prolonged fever, nausea, vomiting, muscle pains, headache, loose cough, confusion, drowsiness and unconsciousness; sometimes also anaemia, yellowness, low blood sugar, and shock. Mental and general symptoms should guide you to the choice of remedy in severe cases, helping you choose between Stramonium, Hyoscyamus, Belladonna and Opium. It is possible that sometimes one of the other remedies already mentioned for the less serious (benign malaria) is indicated, so check them too.

Belladonna

The chill begins in both arms and is without thirst. There is a violent bursting headache and the pupils are dilated; they are worse for light and worse for noise. The face is pale when lying down and red when sitting up. With the heat there is great thirst, and they are much worse for uncovering. Sweat is on covered parts only and it may stain sheets yellow. They are irritable, whining, grumpy or really cross. There is no particular periodicity. There is acuteness of all senses. They are better for warmth and worse for draughts. In delirium they may bite, twitch and scream. They are worse for touch, worse for motion, worse lying down and worse looking at bright objects. They are better for bending backwards and better when leaning the head against something.

Stramonium

There is chill without thirst. The chills run down the back as if from cold water, extending over the whole body. They have a red face, hot head and twitching of limbs. They are worse uncovering, worse after a sleep, worse in the dark, worse for touch, better for warmth and better for company. There is icy cold skin with cold sweat. The heat phase is with thirst, redness and sweat together. The sweat stage has thirst and increased appetite. The delirium and twitching are like Belladonna and there is often trembling and convulsions. They are also loquacious and have wild staring eyes. This type is more violent than Hyos. and Opium, although in actual fact they are very frightened, or really terrified. There is increased saliva and dribbling. The fears are of water, mirrors, and shiny things. They are also worse for any suppressed secretions.

Hyoscyamus

Here there is chill without thirst. They are worse at night and have a short dry hacking cough. During the heat there is thirst, dry skin, distended veins, and the heat runs up the back. During the sweat phase, the sweat is much worse and most profuse on the legs. There is difficulty swallowing liquids and a dry mouth. There are delusions of vision. They frequently make grimaces and silly faces. There can be passive muttering as well as possibly explosive outbursts. There may be involuntary urination or stools. They are worse lying down and better sitting. They are better for warmth, worse for touch. The twitching, delirium and convulsions are like Bell. and Stram., although the delirium and stupor are less active and violent than Bell. or Stram. They may be jealous and suspicious, wanting to escape. They talk to imaginary people and have muttering delirium, or can barely be aroused.

Opium

The chill is without thirst followed by a heat phase with deep stuporous sleep, with the mouth open, and twitching limbs. They can have spasms of facial muscles. This is followed by a profuse sweat and desire to uncover. The heat and sweat phase can happen together and the sweat does not relieve. The appetite is gone. There is profound stupor and unconsciousness, dullness and coma (or sometimes they may be loquacious instead). They are worse for suppressions of secretions, such as sweat, urine, or any discharge. They have trembling, twitching and spasms. They are usually totally constipated. They are much better for cool air and uncovering.

To differentiate between these four remedies, Bell. and Stram. are much more energetically ill and sometimes in extremes are much more violent. Opium is the most comatose, Hyos. is in between and an important keynote for this remedy is making silly faces and grimaces. All the remedies can be delirious. All remedies should be given in a 30 but you may need to go up to a 200 very soon or even start with a 200 if there is already delirium. You could also find you need to go up to a 10M or higher, particularly with Bell. or Stram. if they are being very energetic in their delirium. Improvement should be within minutes if not seconds of giving the remedy; whenever symptoms return you should repeat the remedy. Repetition may be quite frequent particularly at first, see section 10, 'Rules about dosage, potencies and repetition of doses'.

48. Travel sickness

Children usually grow out of travel sickness as they get older but it can occasionally remain a problem into adult life, or return just during pregnancy. One of the three remedies below should help when treating acute symptoms. All three remedies are worse for the motion of a car, boat, bus or aeroplane. If this is a constant problem constitutional treatment from a professional homoeopath should be sought so as to avoid getting sick in the first place.

Tabacum

The main symptoms that would indicate Tabacum are that the sufferer wants to sit wrapped up warm but with his head virtually out of the car window in order to breathe in gulps of fresh air. Fresh air makes Tabacum types feel a lot better and usually seems to prevent actual vomiting; they also want to keep their eyes shut so as not to be looking at moving objects. If they are at sea they want to be on deck (but wrapped up warm) whatever the weather is like, because they must have fresh air. They may be covered in cold sweat and look very pale and pinched. They may also be gloomy and weepy or excitable, talkative and restless.

Cocculus

Cocculus types do not want fresh air but want to remain inside, not moving in the slightest way. They are much worse if they are tired from loss of sleep. At sea you find them lying down on the bunk facing the wall not daring to move an inch. They are better sitting or lying quite still, worse kneeling, stooping or bending, worse for extremes of heat and cold, very much worse for noise, and worse from lack of sleep. If there are no strong indications for either of the other two remedies, this remedy is more often indicated for seasickness.

Petroleum

Symptoms that would indicate Petroleum are that patients are worse from the smell of petrol, do not crave fresh air, prefer dry weather and warmth, and are definitely a lot more irritable than the other two remedies.

DOSAGE

Sometimes you see all three remedies sold as a mixture in health food shops. Although these pills work up to a point, the correct individual homoeopathic remedy works much better on its own. It will take effect faster and only a very few doses are required (quite often only one dose is necessary). Give the remedy as soon as symptoms commence and repeat whenever the symptoms return; a 6 or a 30 is usually all that is required.

49. Long journeys and jet lag

Long journeys can be extremely trying especially for children, as they get tired and irritable. You can prevent a great deal of this by giving Arnica 6 or 12 four-hourly from the beginning of a long journey until you arrive at your destination. It is particularly helpful for people sitting around in airports when flights are delayed and journeys prolonged. When flying you should make sure you drink plenty of water so as to prevent dehydration, which is one of the reasons people become very tired. It is important not to drink alcohol when flying as this increases the dehydration and often is the cause of irrational behaviour when flying. You should find that by following this advice, as well as by taking the Arnica, there should be little or no jet lag.

50. Flying and deep vein thrombosis

Recently there has been an increased awareness of this problem and one cause is thought to be sitting in the cramped conditions of an aeroplane for very long journeys. You can reduce the risk of getting deep vein thrombosis from long flights by buying a mixture of Crataegus Ø with Arnica 6x and with Kali Mur. 6x. You should get it as a liquid remedy mixed up in the proportions of two parts Crataegus Ø, to one part Arnica 6x and one part Kali Mur. 6x. The dose should be 10 drops every hour throughout the flight (unless you are sleeping) and continue for about as many hours after landing as the length of time of the flight itself. The Arnica 6x will also help with any jet lag, see above. There are also the other practical things you must do to minimize any risk, such as wearing support tights and remembering to get up and walk around regularly, or to do foot and ankle exercises from time to time throughout the flight. Those on the contraceptive pill, HRT, or who have had surgery recently, particularly abdominal, are more at risk. Remember that if you are taking any ordinary medication for something else, it may well make the homoeopathic remedies less effective. If you know or fear that you could be at risk anyway, it would be a good idea to consult a professional homoeopath. Proper homoeopathic constitutional treatment should increase your health generally, as well as enable you to get advice about which other acute remedies may help you for this condition. There are many to choose from such as Arsen. Album, Apis, Natrum Sulph., Vipera, Secale, Bothrops, Calc. Ars., Carbo Veg., Hamamelis and others.

51. Care of remedies when travelling

Care of homoeopathic remedies is particularly important when travelling. Remedies should not go through the X-ray machines used for security at airports. There has been a lot of argument about whether or not the X-rays damage homoeopathic remedies. I think the controversy arises because people are unaware that X-ray damage can be cumulative, and that people often have their special homoeopathic travel kits with them; the more frequently the remedies go through the X-ray machine the less effective they become. Most of the remedies people have in their travel kits are usually in a 30C potency or higher and therefore more likely to be susceptible to damage than the lower potencies; (from about a 6C downwards, the potencies may contain some material particle of the original substance so these potencies may be less vulnerable and less likely to be damaged). The remedies will become less and less effective over time as they get more and more zapped by the X-ray machines. It is essential that you can be totally confident in the efficacy of your remedies. There are plenty of situations when serious conditions as well as minor illnesses, could become very painful, unpleasant or dangerous, if left untreated. Being left untreated is in effect what happens when one takes remedies which cannot work because they are damaged (in this case by the X-rays); there may be times when it could even be a matter of life or death. Therefore do **not** be bullied into letting them go through the X-ray machine because some airport official tells you to do so. The airport officials are not homoeopaths and may well have been told that X-rays can do no harm. They will not understand about the difference between the very low potencies and the higher potencies; they will not necessarily realize that people have the same kit which they take with them wherever they travel, so that X-ray damage cumulates; nor will they know that homoeopathy can be used for treating really serious conditions and may well be used to save life. Recently a federal judge in California ruled that two airlines pay a total of $170,000 compensation to the family of someone who died in 1997 because she did not have her allopathic medicines for asthma with her. The airport officials had forbidden her to keep the medicines in her hand luggage and they subsequently were lost or mislaid and unavailable when she needed them. With homoeopathy it is essential to be able to rely on the remedies and we cannot do so if they are zapped by X-rays. The cost of a decent kit of homoeopathic remedies is not cheap and you should not be expected constantly to be replacing them simply to please airport officials. Mostly I have found the security officials perfectly reasonable and helpful. Once I came across a security official who held up the whole queue of travellers while he asked my advice for homoeopathic treatment for his whole family! This was not quite what I expected at 4.30 am on the first day of my holiday, but at least he was enthusiastic about homoeopathy. However, there have been times when they have been very bossy and tiresome, insisting they knew about homoeopathy when they did not, and it has been quite a battle to stop them putting the remedies through the X-ray. Another thing to consider is that if an aircraft flies over about 35,000 feet it is thought that there could possibly be some slight risk of solar radiation damaging the remedies, although this is by no means certain. The best way to avoid the possibility of this problem is to buy a small lead-lined bag from a photographic shop (the ones used to protect films from X-ray damage) and put your remedies in the lead-lined bag in your hand luggage. When you come to the security check at the airport take them out of the lead-lined bag and hand them to the official telling them they have to be checked without going through the X-ray machine. You must do this because if you leave them in the luggage in the lead-lined bag, the security official will simply turn up the dial until the X-ray is strong enough to see through the lead-lined bag. Do not pack them with your main luggage because you never will know whether or not that has been X-rayed. If it has been, the dial will have been turned up until the X-ray was strong enough to see through the lead-lined bag. Currently you can also buy these bags from a mail order company called TravelSmith. Their telephone number in the UK is 0800 783 3030. They do three different sizes and the smallest one would also be useful for the few emergency remedies you might want to keep in your bag to protect them from radiation from your and other people's mobile phones.

While on the subject of X-ray damage, it is worth knowing that a good way of counteracting to some extent the damage done by X-rays to people is to take one dose of X-ray 30 or one dose of Rad. Brom. 30, before and after any X-ray with a final dose at bedtime that evening. This is thought to reduce to some extent the cumulative damage from having any X-rays. (For people who are having radiation therapy as part of their cancer treatment it is best to go to a professional homoeopath to get more specific homoeopathic help.)

You can also buy a laminated Multilingual Travel Card from

Helios Pharmacy which explains in nine different languages about taking care of homoeopathic remedies. I have found this very useful when travelling.

Chapter Six
MATERIA MEDICA

This chapter gives a short Materia Medica (see page 4, Provings) of the remedies used most often in this book. This Materia Medica outlines the *essential characteristics only* of the remedies and gives the detail necessary only for the type of acute ailments I have covered. It is useful for checking to see if you have chosen the most similar remedy when prescribing, as well as a guide if you find yourself treating other minor acute ailments not mentioned in this book. For instance someone who had been on one of my courses gave her son Belladonna 6 for an acutely inflamed toe caused by an ingrowing toenail. We had not mentioned ingrowing toenails during the course but she recognized the symptoms as being the Belladonna remedy picture. These symptoms were very red, hot and swollen, worse for the slightest touch, no pus but the skin being red, shiny and tight with the swelling. While Belladonna does not deal with the chronic symptom of the ingrowing toenail (which would need constitutional treatment), it did cure the acute symptoms very quickly and the toenail did not drop off which it usually had done in the past.

A few homoeopathic remedies are incompatible if given close together. So the two remedies in the following pairs should not precede or follow each other directly.

Causticum and Phosphorus
Silica and Merc. Sol.
Rhus Tox. and Apis
Belladonna and Dulcamara
Dulcamara and Lachesis
Ignatia and Nux Vomica
Ignatia and Tabacum

Aconite

Causes:	Fright; exposure to cold, dry, windy weather.
Main indications:	Acute inflammations, congestions, fevers or colds in the early stages particularly. Hot, burning, red and dry. Fright. Dryness.
Mentals:	Intense fear and restlessness; frantic with fear and/or with the intensity of the pains; anxiety and restlessness with all complaints, even apparently trivial ones. May think they are going to die. (See Arsen. Album.)
Pains:	Intense, burning, tingling, numbness.
Appearance:	Usually robust people when well. In acute has anxious expression, the face may alternate between being pale and red (see Ferrum Phos.), or become very pale on sitting up. One cheek may be hot and red and the other pale (see Chamomilla). Contracted pupils.
Pulse:	Either full and hard or hardly noticeable.
Appetite:	Intense thirst for cold drinks and cold water but preferring bitter drinks such as beer if possible. Worse for milk.
Motion/Position:	Very restless, tosses and turns.
Temperature/ Weather:	Worse for warmth and heat and better uncovering, better for open air and better keeping cool; remember that the acute illness is often caused by exposure to cold, dry, windy weather.
Speed/Time:	Sudden onset always; the early stages of acutes; worse in the evening (about 9 pm particularly) and worse at night.
Touch/Pressure:	Worse touch and pressure.
Sweat/Discharges:	There is extreme dryness running through this remedy picture; dry croupy cough, dry eyes, worse for cold, dry, windy weather, hot, dry inflammations. When the fever breaks they are better for sweating.

Other modalities:	Eyes worse for light and pupils contracted. Generally worse for noise.

Antim. Tart.

Causes:	Damp living conditions.
Main indications:	Particularly indicated during childhood and old age. May be very weak. Great accumulation of mucus in the chest. Cough and pustular eruptions of chickenpox. (Please do not assume that Antim. Tart. is the only homoeopathic remedy for pustular eruptions; there are a great number of remedies for them and as always the remedy must fit the totality of the picture presented by the patient in order to be homoeopathic to the case and to result in cure – also eruptions of any kind are quite often part of a chronic underlying condition which the layperson should not attempt to treat.)
Mentals:	Irritable, easily annoyed or apathetic. Worse for touch but children may cling to those around them and want to be carried. Crying and whining. Cough is worse if the person is angry.
Appearance:	There may be a blue/blackish/grey look around the mouth, lips, nostrils and/or eyes. Tongue usually has a thick white coating with red edges or streaks.
Appetite:	Usually no thirst. Frequently there is nausea which is better for vomiting.
Motion/Position:	Cough better sitting up. Generally worse for motion.
Temperature/ Weather:	Worse spring and autumn, worse for damp, worse for cold, worse overheating.
Speed/Time:	Usually required in later stages of a cough.
Touch/Pressure:	Worse touch.

Sweat/Discharges:	Better for expectoration although this is difficult to raise. Clammy sweat all over.
Other modalities:	Drowsiness and sleepiness with all complaints. Nausea is better for vomiting.

Apis

Causes:	Bites, stings, punctured wounds. Suppressed eruptions.
Main indications:	Puffed up swellings, oedema or swelling like a bag of water.
Mentals:	Fussy about detail, orderly, or clumsy and awkward. Fidgety, restless. Dull, slow, indifferent. Angry if disturbed. Worse alone. Jealous. Stupor, maybe with sudden sharp, shrill cries.
Pains:	Burning and stinging or prickling. Sore, bruised.
Appearance:	Puffiness and swelling of the part; swellings can be transparent or a shiny pinky colour.
Appetite:	Thirstlessness. May desire milk or sour things.
Motion/Position:	Restlessness, cannot keep still, or else completely motionless.
Temperature/ Weather:	Worse for heat, worse for a hot bath, worse for hot drinks, better in cool air and for cool bathing.
Speed/Time:	Sudden onset of symptoms. Worse after sleep.
Touch/Pressure:	Worse for pressure and worse for slightest touch. Head can be better for pressure.
Side:	May be worse on the right side.

Arnica

Causes:	Shock from accidents, injuries, surgery, childbirth. Jet lag.
Main indications:	Shock, whether mild or severe. Bruising. Bleeding internally and externally; passive bleeding, not gushing. Operations.

Mentals:	Fear of approach and/or touch. Insist they are all right even when they obviously are very ill or shocked. May seem dazed and incoherent. May be restless. If delirious answers correctly when spoken to but then returns to unconsciousness at once. Better alone.
Pains:	Sore, bruised, as if beaten.
Appearance:	Bruising, bloodshot, haemorrhage (passive bleeding, not gushing).
Motion/Position:	Restless, tosses and turns. Better lying down, particularly stretched out. Worse for exertion.
Temperature/ Weather:	May have hot head and cold body (particularly during fevers).
Touch/Pressure:	Worse for touch and worse for pressure. Bed feels hard.
Sweat/Discharges:	Smelly sweat, particularly during fevers.
Other modalities:	Worse from noise.

Arsen. Album

Causes:	Eating watery fruit, drinking dirty water or eating dirty vegetables, particularly cold food and drink. Eating bad meat. Overexertion and overheating. High altitudes, lack of oxygen.
Main indications:	Prostration and sinking of strength. Suffering seems out of proportion to the actual symptoms. Vomiting and diarrhoea at the same time.
Mentals:	Extreme anxiety and restlessness. Fastidious, critical and despairing of recovery. Fear of death (Aconite). Cannot stand any kind of disorder. Very much worse alone.
Pains:	Burning pains which are better for heat.
Appearance:	Dry skin, look shrivelled and old, even if they are young. Look deathly pale. Sit hugging the fire as

very much worse for cold, but also will want the window open for fresh air. Sore, red skin from any discharges.

Appetite: Burning thirst but only takes sips at a time; never drinks the whole mug in one go. Craves very cold water which may vomit again immediately; better sips of warm water. Food poisoning usually from eating watery fruits, dirty water or vegetables and occasionally from eating bad meat.

Motion/Position: Extreme restlessness. Better moving and walking about. May even go from bed to bed, or pace up and down.

There is also extreme prostration and exhaustion.

Temperature/ Weather: Cold people, icy cold when ill and better wrapped up and close to the fire. However, they also crave fresh air, so despite being so chilly will insist on having the window wide open with the fire on. Burning pains are also better for heat and hot applications.

Speed/Time: Worse soon after or around midnight and sometimes at midday as well. There is very sudden sinking of strength and prostration, even from fairly trivial causes.

Sweat/Discharges: Any discharges are usually acrid, excoriating and burning and will make the skin sore.

Belladonna

Causes: Exposure to cold, wet weather, getting cold after being hot and sweaty from exertion; exposure to very hot sun; having hair washed and cut.

Main indications: Acute inflammations, congestions or fevers. Heat, burning, swelling, bright redness, shiny, dryness.

Mentals: The mood can be anything from being rather grumpy and hard to please to being furiously angry and quarrelsome, or any stage between these two. They are very restless and oversensitive to all impressions. See monsters when delirious, and can be violent then with shrieking and biting.

Pains: Throbbing, pulsating, spasmodic or cramping.

Appearance: Shiny, bright red, hot and dry inflammations and swellings. Face is fiery red in fever. Pupils dilated. Eyes may be red.

Pulse: Full, hard pulse.

Appetite: Very thirsty, particularly for lemonade or cold water.

Motion/Position: Worse for motion, worse for jarring, worse letting the affected part hang down. Very restless. Worse lying, better sitting propped or bending head backwards.

Temperature/ Weather: Worse for cold, worse uncovering, worse for draughts, better in warm room, better for closed windows. Onset from exposure to cold, wet, windy weather as well as from hot sun.

Speed/Time: Worse about 3 am or 3 pm. Sudden onset. Pains may come and go suddenly.

Touch/Pressure: Worse for slightest touch and worse for pressure.

Sweat/Discharges: While the patient appears very hot, red and dry, there will be dampness and sweat under the hair (particularly the back of the head against the pillow) and under the clothes.

Side: Symptoms worse on right side, or symptoms only on the right side (but this does not mean the symptoms are never on the left side).

Other modalities: Worse for the slightest noise. Hypersensitive. While there is terrific heat, dryness and redness throughout this remedy picture there is also sweat and dampness under the hair and clothing, particularly during the fevers.

Bryonia

Causes:	Exposure to cold, dry, windy weather; eating cold food or drink when overheated or in very hot weather; financial worries; suppressed sweats or skin eruptions.
Main indications:	Dryness of all mucous membranes; inflammations and exudation (the oozing of fluid into a cavity/organ).
Mentals:	Better when alone and worse for company. Irritable, taciturn. Worried about job, business or homework. Sounds resentful and accusing. If delirious talk about their work or job and want to go home even if they are at home.
Pains:	Sharp stitching pains; soreness.
Appearance:	Dark red, congested, bloated looking face. Lips extremely dry, patient licks them to moisten them, which only makes them worse. Any local swellings are pale red.
Pulse:	Hard and hurried.
Appetite:	Extremely thirsty for cold and warm drinks; drinks a lot at a time; drinks hurriedly; worse for warm drinks; worse for rich, fatty, greasy food.
Motion/Position:	Pains are very much worse for slightest motion (although you may find that the pain drives them to restlessness despite the fact that this aggravates it). Worse for being jarred.
Temperature/ Weather:	Worse for hot weather, better for cool open air. Worse cooling down suddenly when hot.
Touch/Pressure:	Worse for light touch but better for firm pressure.
Speed/Time:	Onset is slow, over a few days rather than hours. May be worse at about 9 pm.
Sweat/Discharges:	This is a very dry remedy where sweat, discharges or eruptions have been suppressed.
Side:	Mostly left-sided.

Calendula

Main indications:	To stop haemorrhages (undiluted Ø). Use with water to clean wounds. As a lotion or cream for burns, cuts, scratches. To prevent sepsis; may need to alternate with Hypericum for this. Episiotomy.
Appearance:	For bleeding, use undiluted Ø. Cuts, scratches, burns.
Sweat/Discharges:	Haemorrhage.

Chamomilla

Causes:	Teething. Anger. Pain.
Main indications:	Extreme bad temper and irritability with any pain. Particularly useful during teething, both for the pains and for diarrhoea.
Mentals:	Furious anger with any pain, adults can seem extremely bad-tempered, but it is due to the pain. Babies are capricious, throwing away whatever they have just demanded. They are better for being carried and walked up and down. They fight and throw themselves around as well as scream if you try to put them back into the cot.
Pains:	Intolerable. Sweat and heat with pain. Numbness may follow the pains. Anger with the pains.
Appearance:	One cheek red and the other pale. One side hot and red and the other cool and pale. One half of the body is hot and red while the other is cool and pale; either the front and back, or top half and bottom half.
Appetite:	Desires and is better for cold drinks and very much worse for hot drinks. Thirst for cold water. Increased saliva.
Motion/Position:	Better for being carried particularly if carried and walked up and down, worse lying in bed or cot, worse being put down into the cot.

Temperature/ Weather:	Generally hot. Teething and gum pains are worse for warm food and worse for warm drink, but stomach pains and colic better for warmth.
Touch/Pressure:	Worse for touch.
Sweat/Discharges:	Hot sweat with pains.
Side:	One-sided pains, heat and redness.

Drosera

Causes:	Whooping cough.
Main indications:	Incessant cough. Paroxysms of coughing. Whooping cough.
Mentals:	Easily angry. Worse alone.
Motion/Position:	Worse lying down.
Temperature/ Weather:	Better fresh open air. Worse for warmth and heat.
Speed/Time:	Worse after midnight to about 3 am.
Touch/Pressure:	Better pressure.

Dulcamara

Causes:	Exposure to cold, wet weather, or sudden changes from hot, dry weather to cold, wet weather. Autumn. Cooling down suddenly when hot and sweaty.
Main indications:	Any complaints from getting chilled particularly when already hot and sweaty.
Mentals:	Impatient, scolding, bossy. Make mountains out of molehills.
Pains:	Pinching, cutting, griping pains with diarrhoea; particularly around the navel.
Motion/Position:	Better for motion.
Temperature/ Weather:	Worse from sudden temperature changes particularly from hot and dry to cold and wet. Worse cooling down when hot and sweaty. Worse

for warm days and cold nights. Worse in the
autumn. Better warm and dry.

Speed/Time: Generally worse at night.

Ferrum Phos.

Causes: Cold, checked sweat, mechanical injuries.

Main indications: Local congestions; early stages of fevers, colds and
                     inflammations. This remedy is not as
                     'energetically' sick as Belladonna and Aconite nor
                     as sluggish and lethargic as Gelsemium. It lies
                     somewhere between the two extremes.
                     Symptoms can seem rather nondescript.
                     Weakness and prostration.

Mentals: Dissatisfied or indifferent even to nice things,
                     occasionally excitable; may alternate these moods.
                     Averse to company usually.

Pains: Bruised soreness.

Appearance: Alternate between being flushed and pale. Any
                     local swellings are pale not red. When well usually
                     appear pale. Bleeds easily; bloodshot eyes.

Appetite: Worse for warm drinks better for cold drinks.
                     No appetite, or eats without enjoying it.

Motion/Position: Better gentle motion, worse for exertion. Better
                     lying down. Worse for being jarred.

Temperature/   Worse for cold. Desires fresh air and is worse in
Weather: stuffy rooms. Local congestions and flushes of
                     heat. Usually a cold person.

Speed/Time: The early stages of acute inflammations and
                     fevers. May be worse at night. Usually symptoms
                     come on quite fast.

Sweat/Discharges: Discharges are blood-streaked. Ill effects of
                     checked sweat. Bleeds easily.

Other modalities: Worse for noise.

Gelsemium

Causes:	Hot climates, heat of sun, summer. Damp, hot, humid weather. Temporary anticipatory fears.
Main indications:	Aching, weakness and tremors. Heaviness, drowsiness, lack of muscular co-ordination, even paralysis. Fevers accompanied by these symptoms.
Mentals:	Nervousness; temporary anticipatory fears. Shaking, trembling with fear. Better alone, does not want anyone near them even if they are silent. Apathetic. Dazed.
Pains:	Aching, heaviness, soreness.
Appearance:	Shaking, trembling. Drooping eyelids. Hands tremble.
Pulse:	Slow, weak pulse.
Appetite:	No thirst even during heat of fever. May become thirsty during sweat. Dry mouth and lips but no thirst.
Motion/Position:	Worse for motion generally because of the extreme weakness. Worse for downward motion. Better continuous gentle motion. Better sitting propped up particularly when they have a headache.
Temperature/ Weather:	Generally worse for heat. Worse in humid, damp, hot weather. Hot head with cold body. Shivers of cold run up and down spine, despite being hot and sweaty.
Touch/Pressure:	Desires to be held when shivering and shaking.
Speed/Time:	Slow onset.
Sweat/Discharges:	Better for profuse urination, particularly the headache. Generally better for sweating.

Hepar Sulph.

Causes:	Exposure to cold, dry winds.

Main indications:	Tendency to suppuration. Early stages of suppuration, before pus has formed and in the early stages once pus has formed. Oversensitive mentally and physically. Sluggishness with weak expulsive power. Smelly discharges.
Mentals:	Oversensitive to pain and all impressions. Touchy. Quarrelsome, irritable, dissatisfied. Hasty and impulsive.
Pains:	Sticking pains like sharp splinters.
Appetite:	Desires sharp stimulating tastes such as vinegar, acids and pickles. Drinks hastily.
Temperature / Weather:	Chilly person, worse for cold, dry winds. Worse for draughts and better for closed windows. Better for damp weather, particularly with coughs and croup.
Touch/Pressure:	Worse for slightest touch and pressure. Worse lying on affected part.
Speed/Time:	Worse at night particularly the early hours of the morning from about 5 am. Early stages of pus formation, later stages of colds.
Sweat/Discharges:	Thick or thin but pustular discharges. Sweat and all discharges smell sour.

Hypericum

Main indications:	Injuries to parts rich in nerves, such as the fingertips or the spine. To prevent sepsis and tetanus (alternate with Ledum). Bites, stings and punctured wounds. As a cream or lotion for burns. As a cream or lotion for cuts, grazes, and lacerated wounds.
Pains:	Travel up the limb from the injury.
Appearance:	Red streaks running up the limb from the injury.
Motion/Position:	Worse for motion.
Temperature / Weather:	Worse for cold.

Touch/Pressure: Worse for touch.

Ipecac.

Causes: Overeating rich food. Suppressed eruptions. Teething. Vexation, reserved displeasure; particularly if people think they have been treated or punished unfairly.

Main indications: Coughs with profuse mucus in the lungs which is hard to raise. Bleeding bright red blood. Persistent nausea with any complaint; no better for vomiting. Clean tongue. Fermented stools, grass green stools or slimy stools.

Mentals: Capricious. Irritable. Sulky. Cannot stomach insults.

Pains: Nausea with every pain.

Appearance: Clean tongue always despite the constant nausea. Saliva increased.

Appetite: Thirstless. Worse overeating rich foods. Constant nausea no better for vomiting.

Motion/Position: Better sitting. Worse for motion.

Temperature/
Weather: Worse for damp weather. Better for fresh air.

Sweat/Discharges: Easily haemorrhages, bright red blood.

Side: Sometimes may have one red cheek (Chamomilla).

Other modalities: Vomiting without any relief from it.

Ledum

Main indications: Punctured wounds, bites of any kind, stings, splinters. Tetanus (alternate with Hypericum).

Pains: Shooting, pricking pains.

Appearance: Purple, puffy/dropsical swellings.

Temperature/ Weather:	Parts are cold to the touch although they may feel hot to the patient. Better for cold bathing, better for cool air, better for ice cold water, better uncovering, worse for warmth.
Touch/Pressure:	Worse for any touch.

Nux Vomica

Causes:	Overeating rich food. Hangovers. Sedentary habits. Stimulants such as coffee, alcohol, drugs, cigarettes.
Main indications:	Oversensitivity to all impressions. Headache or breathing problems with every gastric upset; usually from overeating and drinking.
Mentals:	Self-reliant, ambitious, efficient, conscientious, hardworking people but who are also impatient, aggressive, irritable and short-tempered. Angry, fiery temperament worse for consolation. Always feel irritable inside.
Pains:	Angry, impatient with the pain. Cannot stand the pain.
Appearance:	Thin, spare active people usually.
Appetite:	Ailments from overeating and drinking too much. Desire stimulants, alcohol, rich food.
Temperature/ Weather:	Chilly people, worse for cold, worse for wind, worse for draughts. Better wrapped and better covered up. Better for wet and rainy weather rather than dry weather.
Touch/Pressure:	Worse for touch and worse for pressure.
Speed/Time:	Worse first thing in the morning.
Sweat/Discharges:	Smelly breath.
Other modalities:	Urge to stool with every pain. Twitchings and jerkings with symptoms.

Phosphorus

Causes: Exposure to very heavy rain, weather change, going from hot to cold atmosphere or from cold to hot, eating too much salt, putting hands into very cold water; anaesthetic.

Main indications: Exhausting diarrhoea; lung problems with weight on chest sensation; haemorrhages; nervous exhaustion; always wants company; burning pains.

Mentals: Excitable and impressionable. Fears to be alone, fears the dark, fears thunder. Loves company, wants to go to the party however ill they are. Sympathetic and loves sympathy.

Pains: Tightness in chest; weight on chest. Burning pains.

Appearance: Tall and slim.

Appetite: Worse for too much salt, desires salt. Desires and is better for cold food and drink, but vomits almost immediately as it warms in stomach; worse for warm food and drink.

Motion/Position: Worse lying on left side, or on back or painful side, better lying on right side.

Temperature/ Weather: Worse from thunderstorms and lightning; worse warm food and drink; worse from change of weather and change of room temperature. Cold relieves head and face symptoms but worsens cough, and sore throats. Generally chilly people.

Speed/time: Particularly worse at dusk.

Touch/Pressure: Desires massage.

Sweat/Discharges: Bloody. Bleeds very easily, bright red blood.

Pulsatilla

Main indications: Changeable symptoms, both physically and mentally. Pains move around and change from place to place; the type of pains change. Moods change easily from tears to laughter and back again. Thick discharges. Digestive upsets. Dependant.

Mentals: Weepy, tearful mood. Worse alone. Affectionate. Mild, gentle, timid people usually. Easily moved to laughter or to tears. Changeable mood.

Pains: Start gradually but stop suddenly. Pains wander around from place to place, constantly changing. Relieved by cool.

Appetite: Worse eating rich foods, such as pastry or cream, although these are liked and desired. Dislikes pork. Wants refreshing foods. Worse for greasy foods, worse for warm foods. Thirstlessness, even with a dry mouth.

Motion/Position: Better moving gently. Better changing positions. Worse lying on left side particularly. Better sitting upright.

Temperature/ Weather: Usually warm people; they are worse overheating and can overheat easily. Very much worse for stuffy rooms, desire fresh air. With any pains or during any illness can become cold, although they are usually warm. Better for cool applications.

Speed/Time: Worse in the evenings.

Touch/Pressure: Better for touch and pressure. Babies and children particularly want cuddles. May be clingy.

Sweat/Discharges: Profuse, bland thick discharges. Usually yellowish-green or creamy coloured; frequently changeable in appearance.

Rhus Tox.

Causes: Exposure to cold, wet and damp weather. Cooling down suddenly after being hot and sweaty. Injuries from overexertion. Draughts.

Main indications:	Muscular pains from overexertion or from fevers, flu. Itchy eruptions of chickenpox. Strained muscles and stiffness. Torn ligaments and tendons particularly if near joints; sprains. It is specifically indicated for ankle injuries.
Mentals:	Extreme restlessness with all complaints. Despair about their pain. Forget what they have just asked for. Very sad and despondent.
Pains:	Tearing, bruised, soreness. Feeling of dislocation. Itching of chickenpox.
Appearance:	Triangular red tip to an otherwise coated tongue; or else diagonally/half coated while the rest is bright red.
Appetite:	Thirsty for cold drinks particularly cold milk. Not much appetite.
Motion/Position:	Restless and generally better for motion. Pains worse for initial movement, better for continued motion and worse for hard exertion. Worse for rest and when still.
Temperature/ Weather:	Worse for exposure to cold, damp, wet weather and draughts. Worse uncovering. Better for a hot bath and wrapping up warm. Better for dry warmth. Worse cooling down suddenly when hot and sweaty.
Touch/Pressure:	Better rubbing painful parts. Better lying on something hard.
Speed/Time:	Slow onset. Symptoms return at same hour day after day.
Sweat/Discharges:	May have urticaria during fever, which gets better at the onset of sweating.
Side:	May be mostly left-sided, or start at the left and spread to the right side (Lach.).

Ruta

Main indications: Bruised, wrenched, torn tendons. Kicks and knocks to periosteum. Sports injuries involving these parts. Following osteopathic treatments. Nodes, nodules, bursae, ganglion. It is specifically indicated for wrist injuries.

Symphytum

Main indications: Injuries to eyeball, cheek bone and bones surrounding the eye. Broken or cracked bones.

APPENDICES

1. Buying homoeopathic remedies

There are various homoeopathic pharmacies which supply homoeopathic remedies through the post. Usually the service is very efficient and
if you tell them it is urgent you will probably get the remedy the next
day. However, it is a good idea to have a supply at home of the remedies
you think you may need most. Some of the more common remedies you
can get from health food shops and the brand names to look out for are
Nelsons or Weleda; these remedies are nearly always in a 6C potency,
although sometimes now a 30C is available. Remedies should remain
potent forever, providing they are not antidoted, see section 8.

**The following is a list of reliable homoeopathic pharmacies
in the UK that send remedies out by post:**

Helios Homoeopathic Pharmacy,
89-97 Camden Road, Royal Tunbridge Wells, TN1 2QR.
Tel: 01892-536393. E-mail pharmacy@helios.co.uk

Ainsworths Homoeopathic Pharmacy,
36 New Cavendish Street, London, W1G 8UF.
Tel: 020-7935-5330.

Galen Homoeopathics,
Lewell Mills, West Stafford, Dorchester, DT2 8AN.
Tel: 01305-263996.

Prices of remedies vary, as do the sizes of the bottles and the types of
pills. I think Helios's 4 gm bottle of pillules which contains about 100
pillules is very good value. Helios is also happy to make up first aid kits
to your own specification, consisting of ten remedies in the 4gm size
or the 5 ml liquid size. For very young babies you may prefer liquid
remedies or else the larger soft tablets (but then you do not get so

many per bottle). The advantage of these kits is that it is then easy to find the correct remedy in an emergency; this is highly preferable to wasting precious time by wading through bags full of remedies from different pharmacies or health food shops, trying to find a particular remedy. You can make up as many first aid kits as you like but you must remember to specify the potency required, whether you want pillules, tablets, soft tablets, powders or a liquid, the size of the bottle as well as the name and potency of the remedy. Despite what may be written on the remedy labels of brands found in health food shops, one pill or tablet (not two) is enough for a homoeopathic dose of any potency above a 6C. Helios also provide a 'Basics Kit' Reference DH18 which contains 18 remedies in 2mg size bottles of pillules; and a 'Basics Plus Kit' Reference DH36 which contains the 18 remedies of the DH18 kit plus another 18 remedies; both kits come with a very brief instruction leaflet.

2. Other useful addresses

The Homoeopathic Supply Company,
The Street, Bodham, Holt, Norfolk, NR25 6AD, UK.
Tel: 01263–588788. E-mail: orders@homeopathicsupply.com
   They supply cases for homoeopthic remedies, bottles and other useful items.

TravelSmith,
Freepost EX151, Exeter, EX 124, UK.
Tel: 0800 783 3030.
   They are a mail order company for travel items and supply X-ray film bags. These are lead-lined bags and are very useful for preventing damage to homoeopathic remedies from radiation. The bags currently come in three sizes, 7"x 5", 8" x 9.5" and 12" x 10.5". The smallest is suitable for keeping a few remedies safe from mobile phone damage in your bag, and the other two can hold a variety of remedy containers and similarly protect them, see page 25.

3. Qualified homoeopaths and how to find them

The Society of Homoeopaths is the professional body for practising classical homoeopaths. It has a Register, which lists the names and addresses of all properly qualified homoeopaths in the UK. (It also has a few homoeopaths listed in Australia, Canada, France, Hong Kong, Iceland, Kenya, New Zealand, Saudi Arabia, Singapore, United Arab Emirates, USA and the West Indies.) These homoeopaths have done a training of at least four years in a college whose prospectus and standards reach those agreed by the Society. The Society's aims include developing and maintaining high standards for the practice of homoeopathy. If you are in any doubt about the qualifications of homoeopaths the first question to ask is how long their training was and the second is whether they are on the Register of The Society of Homoeopaths. If they are on the Register they are allowed to use the letters RSHom. after their name. The Society of Homoeopaths is happy to give you the names of local homoeopaths and it can be contacted at: The Society of Homoeopaths, 2 Artizan Road, Northampton, NN1 4HU, UK. Tel: 01604-621400.

4. BSE enquiry

BSE, or bovine spongiform encephalopathy, is a disease of cattle which is related to Crutzfeldt-Jakob disease, CJD, in humans.

At the BSE enquiry, Statement of information number 483 reported the concerns Sir Richard Southwood had had in 1988 about the transmission of BSE to humans via medicinal products, particularly transmission via vaccinations. The enquiry quoted Dr. Pickles as saying that those most at risk from infection with the BSE agent were those receiving medical products of bovine origin: also that inoculation posed a much greater risk of transmission of BSE than the oral route. It was pointed out that sensible precautions were taken to exclude the use of tissues and fluids from scrapie-infected animals, using those only from clinically well animals. This however, was not considered sufficient protection as far as BSE was concerned because it was not possible to determine which animals were infected, particularly in view of the apparently long incubation period, and the fact that infection can be present without actual clinical disease.

The Licensing Authority and the Committee on Safety of Medicines had been made aware of the risks and eventually they had reassured Sir Richard Southwood that appropriate precautions were being put in place as well as additional guidance being given to medicine manufacturers on good manufacturing practice. In view of this action, the risk of infecting humans with BSE via inoculation from then on, (1989) was described as 'remote'. The BSE enquiry has shown the potential risk of transmission of BSE via inoculation since actions taken in 1989 to be remote, but before 1989 the potential risk could have been relatively high.

It is extremely disturbing that those vaccines which still had some years of shelf life left, were not immediately withdrawn and destroyed after the conclusions were reached in 1989; it was considered that such action would have caused public alarm. Instead, over the next few years they were supposed to have been used up and gradually replaced by vaccines made under the new guidelines. It seems incredible that parents were not told about this at the time. Surely parents should have been informed that their choice between vaccination and non-vaccination at that time was in fact a choice between the risk, however slight, of their child contracting BSE/CJD, or having the childhood diseases; a choice between a killer disease with no cure whatsoever, or childhood diseases which can be successfully treated with homoeopathic medicine, common sense and generally good living standards.

It is time that the vaccination history of all those people who so tragically have died of BSE/CJD, or are currently suffering from it, be examined. This could be particularly significant as those most affected are the young, who are also those who have been most frequently vaccinated. It could also be one of the possible contributory factors for the high incidence of the disease in certain areas; perhaps the victims all had their vaccinations from a small number of contaminated batches. Surely the reason vaccines and medicines have reference numbers and batch numbers is so that if there is a disaster they can then be traced.

One hopes the new guidelines are being followed, but reports such as the one in *The New York Times* on 8 February 2001, indicating that a number of companies making vaccines were still using materials from cattle from BSE-infected countries in 2000, are very disturbing. It is now over ten years since the possible dangers were known, yet such reports suggest that there is apparently still a possibility of potentially contaminated bovine products being used in our vaccines. One wonders how many people have had vaccines which were suspect in the interim.

5. Further reading

Blackie, Margery G., *The Patient not the Cure*, Macdonald and Jane's, 1976.

Chaitow, Leon, *Vaccination and Immunization*, C.W. Daniel Co. Ltd., 1987.

Chancellor, Philip M., *Handbook of the Bach Flower Remedies*, C.W. Daniel Co. Ltd., 1971.

Coulter, Harris, *Homoeopathic Science and Modern Medicine*, North Atlantic Books, 1981.

Coulter, Harris and Fisher, Barbara, *DPT: A Shot in the Dark*, Harcourt Brace Jovanovich, 1985.

Shepherd, Dorothy, *Magic of the Minimum Dose*, Health Science Press, 1974.

Vitoulkas, George, *The Science of Homoeopathy*, Grove Press Inc., 1980.

Crook, Alan, *A Christian's Guide to Homoeopathy*, Winter Press, 1996.

INDEX

Page numbers written in **bold** refer to the pages where there is a detailed remedy picture description or prescribing instructions for that particular remedy, not just a reference to that particular remedy.

HOMOEOPATHY: THE MODERN PRESCRIBER

Gum abscess   110, 111, 112, 113

Haemorrhage   45, 53, 195, 199, 204, 206
Hahnemann   2–5, 7–9 ,18, 21
Handling homoeopathic remedies 23–25
Hangovers   105, 205
Headaches   74, 113–117, 123
Head lice   113, 123
Hepar Sulph.   **50**, 53, 74, 76, **79**, 80–86, **89**, **90**, **95**, 97–103, **112**, 113, **202**, **203**
Hippocrates   3
Homoeopathic pharmacist/ Pharmacies   21, 47, 211, 212
Homoeopathic remedies:
  care of and when taking them 23–25
  dosage   30–34
  how they are made   21–22
  how to choose   25–30
  where to buy   211
Homoeopaths, how to find qualified ones   213
Housemaid's knee   43
Hypericum   **44**, **46**, 47, **48**, 49, 50, 51, 52, 53, **54**, 55, 57, 58, 59, 60, 61, **80**, **112**, 199, **203**, **204**
Hyoscyamus   182, **183**, 184

Ignatia   **41**, 191
Immunization/inoculation/ vaccination, damage from 125–131, 166, 213, 214, 216
Improvement, signs of, in acutes 33–36
Inherited weaknesses, miasms   7, 18, 37
Insecticides   123

Insect stings/bites   54–57
Ipecac.   **95**, 96, 97–103, **105**, 106, 108, 111, **142**, 144, **157**, **180**, **204**

Jelly fish stings   54, 56
Jet lag   186–187, 194
Journeys   186–187

Kali Bich.   78, 82, 83, 85, **96**, 97–102, **116**, **142**, 143, **144**, 149, 153, 154
Kali Mur.   **187**
Kicks and knocks   43, 53, 209
Knife wounds   47

Lac Can.   **150**, 153–155
Lacarated wounds   52–53, 203
Lachesis   **137**, **150**, 152–155, 191, 208
Lavender   123
Lathyrus Sativus   **160**, **162**
Law of similars   3, 4, 125
Ledum   **43**, **48**, **51**, 52, 53, **54**, 55, 57, 60, **112**, 203, **204**
Lice   113, 123, 124
Lice solution   123, 124
Ligaments, torn   44, 208
Ligature   45, 46, 56
Limb, loss of, pain in stump   44
Lotions (see also Dressings)   45, 46, 123, 132, 133
Lycopodium   **137**, **150**, 152–156

Mag. Phos.   **109**, **110**
Malaria, the disease   3, 173, 178–179
Malaria, prevention of disease 174, 175, 176, 177, 178
Malaria, treatment of disease 178–184